BUILT TO LAST AFTER 50

The truth about **arthritis, strength,** and **staying independent**

PHIL EVANS

Phil the Physio

Rethink

First published in Great Britain in 2026
by Rethink Press (www.rethinkpress.com)

Cover image © Shutterstock / Valenty

Chapter 1 image credits: Quadriceps – Shutterstock / KNEEguru; Glutes – Shutterstock / Stocktrek Images

Disclaimer

The information provided in this book is for educational and informational purposes only and is not intended as medical advice. It is not a substitute for professional diagnosis, treatment, or advice from a qualified healthcare provider. Always seek the advice of your physician or another qualified health professional before making any changes to your medical treatment or health regimen.

The author and publisher disclaim any liability for any loss or damage incurred as a result of the use or misuse of the information contained in this book. No doctor–patient relationship is created by this publication.

Contents

Introduction

If you're over fifty and waking up every morning with stiff, achy joints; or if your muscles feel weaker, no matter how much you keep active; or if everyday things like walking upstairs, carrying shopping, or playing with your grandkids are starting to feel tougher than they should, then this book is for you.

Maybe you've started to dread going on long walks. Maybe you feel nervous about losing your independence, or maybe you even have to say no to your grandchildren, who are desperate for you to play with them.

What about when you finally ask for help? You've been fobbed off with painkillers, told 'It's just your age, what do you expect?', or handed a sheet of generic exercises.

Maybe you've sat on a waiting list for months, even years, for surgery that may not even solve your problem. Perhaps you've spent hours on Google or YouTube, only to end up more confused, unsure who to trust, and worried you'll make things worse.

Sound familiar?

If you've ever caught yourself thinking, *Is this it? Is this how life is going to be from now on?*, keep reading.

Pain and stiffness are not inevitable just because you're getting older; they're simply warning signs that your body is losing strength and capacity. If you ignore this, life starts to shrink. First long walks, then it's stairs. Then maybe family trips. Before you know it, you're living life around pain instead of the way you want.

That's why I wrote this book – to cut through the noise, give you straight answers, and show you steps you can take to avoid decline.

My book is for anyone over fifty who wants to keep living life to the full. It's for the grandparent who wants to stay playful, the retired professional who wants to keep travelling and enjoying life, and the health-conscious individual who refuses to settle for just putting up with it.

It's useful to know which type of person you are. Do you push through, grit your teeth and bear it, pretending nothing's wrong? Do you struggle on, letting pain dictate what you can and can't do? Have you started withdrawing, saying no to things you once loved and watching life shrink around you?

The good news is that no matter which group you're in right now, there's a way forward. This book will show you how to move from coping and struggling to finally regaining control, mobility, and confidence.

Who am I and why should you listen to me?

I'm Phil Evans, a chartered physiotherapist who's spent the last twenty years working in two very different worlds. I started my career in elite sport where I worked with top rugby players, professional cricketers, even with Great Britain judo and bobsleigh teams, and with the Olympic and Commonwealth athletes in preparation for the 2012 London Olympics and the 2014 Commonwealth Games in Glasgow. In that world, nothing is left to chance, nothing is left unturned. These sportspeople got unlimited treatment; they got all the tests that they needed to enable them to perform and stay fit. If they couldn't move, they couldn't play. End of story.

The other world is yours. You're over fifty, your joints hurt, and when you finally pluck up the courage to ask for help, you're fobbed off with a load of painkillers and maybe a printout of exercises that don't fit your life. Then the words no one wants to hear, 'Come back in six months.' In that moment, it feels like you've been dismissed. Like your pain doesn't matter, and your independence and your future aren't urgent enough to fix right now.

That's why I founded my own business, Urban Body, which began in my parents' front room, treating friends and family. Twenty years later, it's an award-winning clinic in Solihull. I've spent my career on the frontline, working with thousands of people over fifty to help them move better, ditch the pills, and get back to the stairs, the walks, and the grandchildren on their terms.

Here's what really frustrated me most with this whole process: the very science and strategies that I learned and used working with elite athletes, to keep them finely tuned and on the pitch, are the exact same ones that could keep *you* active, independent, and free from painkillers. Yet for too long, those solutions have been locked away in the world of sport, while people like you are left waiting, guessing, and losing hope. Since starting Urban Body, I have wanted to bring the best of an elite sport attitude into everyday lives.

Today, Urban Body is more than me. It's a hand-picked team of specialist therapists who put people first, listening, caring, and treating every patient as an individual. What makes us unique is that we combine this person-centred approach with advanced therapies that no other clinic offers under one roof. Treatments once reserved for elite athletes are now being used to help ordinary people in their fifties, sixties, and beyond regain independence, confidence, and joy in life.

My mission is simple: to bring world-class physio care and advanced treatment technologies into private practice for ordinary people who deserve better than a lifetime of painkillers and waiting lists.

What is the real problem?

Let me be clear: I think the NHS is incredible when it comes to serious or life-threatening conditions. We in the UK are so lucky to have it, and I'll always say that. If you have a heart attack, cancer, or a serious infection, there's nowhere in the world you'd rather be.

However, here's the part no one really talks about. The NHS was never designed to provide long-term proactive care for non-life-threatening problems like arthritis, back pain, stiffness, or achy joints. It's a system built to save lives, not to keep you strong, mobile, and independent as you age.

Instead of personalised hands-on treatment, you're offered painkillers, a leaflet of generic exercises, and a place on a waiting list. While you wait (weeks or sometimes months), your muscles get weaker, your confidence drops, and your world gets smaller.

This is what I call the painkiller pandemic, and it's a vicious cycle where pain leads to inactivity, inactivity leads to weakness, weakness makes the joints hurt more, and round it goes. The real problem isn't your arthritis; it isn't just wear and tear; and it certainly isn't inevitable ageing. The problem is a broken system that manages decline instead of preventing it in the first place.

If you want to break that cycle, if you want to become strong and confident and pain-free, you're in the right place. This is what athletes get, and that's what you've been denied until now.

What you'll get from this book

By the end of this book, you'll know exactly what to do (and just as importantly, what not to do) to keep your joints, muscles, and independence strong well into your sixties, seventies, and beyond. You'll get clarity instead of confusion, so there's no more wasting hours on Google or YouTube wondering which exercises are safe. You'll have a clear step-by-step approach that actually works.

You'll learn the truth about arthritis, ageing, and muscle loss. You'll understand why wear and tear isn't the end of the story and how to reverse the decline with the right plan.

I'll share simple, enjoyable routines with you that make movement fun and achievable, not a chore or a one-size-fits-all approach. You'll learn clear movement principles, along with simple example exercises you can safely try at home, plus guidance on how to build them into everyday life without it becoming overwhelming. To remove guesswork, I've put together a simple online hub I call the Vault. You'll find guided videos and examples that show you exactly how things should look and feel. You can access the Vault via the Resources page at the back of the book, by visiting pages.philthephysio.com/vault, or by scanning the QR code below:

You'll gain the confidence to move again. Rebuild trust in your body and stop living in fear of making things worse. Follow a roadmap to get off the pain merry-go-round with natural science-backed ways to reduce pain and restore strength (so you don't have to rely on tablets just to cope).

I'll explain advanced therapies. You'll discover how elite-level treatments like Neubie neuromuscular stimulation, red light therapy, and hyperbaric oxygen can accelerate recovery, reduce pain, and give you an edge.

It's all about staying mobile as you age. Throughout the book, you'll find stories and strategies from real people like you. Proof that it's never too late to turn things around, regain your spark, and enjoy the freedom of living life on your own terms.

How does this book work? The structure is simple. It follows the same process I use in my clinic every day.

Think of it like coaching. You wouldn't expect to win a rugby match by only reading the rule book. You need a strategy, training, and a coach to keep you accountable. This book will give you all three!

Why does this matter? Let me ask you, why have you picked this book up? Is it to play with your grandchildren without wincing? Is it to walk the hills with your partner without worrying about your knees? Is it to feel confident about getting in and out of a chair or a car without grabbing on to something? Or is it something quieter than that, the worry that if things keep sliding, you'll start relying on others? That your world might shrink little by little? That the independence you've worked your whole life for could slowly erode? Whatever your reason, that's your fuel. Write it down, stick it on the fridge, because when life gets busy and excuses creep in, that's what will get you moving again.

Are you ready? Let's get going! Your first step awaits.

1

Finding The Right Cause: Why Guessing Gets You Nowhere

I'll start with something you may already know in your gut: guessing doesn't work. Yet that's exactly what most people do when it comes to their joint pain.

Let me introduce you to Jane. She was in her early sixties, and she came to me when her knees were so sore she could barely manage the stairs in her own house. What struck me wasn't her pain (as unfortunately, I see this all the time). It was the plastic bag that she was carrying. It contained half-empty tubs of turmeric capsules, glucosamine, CBD oils, resistance bands that she'd bought online, and even a knee brace that was still in its box.

She told me that she had tried everything – and she had! Every week, she latched on to the new miracle solution. A YouTube yoga routine, an arthritis diet from a magazine, and advice from a friend at her walking club.

Jane wasn't lazy, and she certainly wasn't unmotivated. In fact, she was one of the most determined women I'd ever met. Nonetheless, her knees were worse than ever, and she was exhausted, demoralised, and quietly terrified that a wheelchair was in her near future.

The truth is, her problem wasn't lack of effort. The problem was guessing.

That's exactly what the system pushes you into. You ask for help, and you're told, 'Take these painkillers, try to stay active, come back in six weeks if it hasn't improved.' That's not a plan, that's guesswork. It's like trying to fix a car engine blindfolded: you jiggle a wire, swap a part, add some oil, hoping something might work. Sometimes the car will splutter along a little bit, but more often than not, the problem gets worse.

That's what happens when people with joint pain are left to guess their way through. When the stakes are this high (ie, your independence, your confidence, your ability to play with your grandchildren, take a holiday, or even just get up the stairs without fear of pain), that's a gamble you can't afford to take.

The real issue is this: too often we treat the symptoms, not the cause. Painkillers can mask discomfort for a few hours, but they don't rebuild strength. A sheet of generic exercises might make you feel like you're doing something, but it won't restore your mobility or confidence.

If you think I'm exaggerating, I'm not. NICE (the organisation that writes the official guidelines for general and healthcare practitioners) also admits it. Their 2021 chronic pain guidance makes it clear that too many people are managed with nothing more than painkillers and generic exercise sheets.[1] They specifically recommend tailored person-centred plans, because pain management has to be built around the individual, not a one-size-fits-all handout.

If you've ever felt like you've been left to figure it out on your own, you're not imagining it. The system really does have you gambling with your independence.

The good news is that there's a better way. You don't need luck; you need a process, and that's what this book is going to give you.

The three types of arthritis patients

Before we go any further, let's make this personal. Most people who pick up this book fall into one of three categories. Think of it like three different drivers on the road and see which one sounds most like you.

Class 1: The Marys

Mary is sixty-five. She's noticed some stiffness in her hips and knees. It's like her car's wheels are spinning on the ground, and there's a yellow warning sign flashing on her dashboard. She hasn't broken down yet, but she knows something's off.

Her general practitioner (GP) told her it's just ageing, gave her painkillers, and advised her to try swimming. Deep down, Mary knows that's not enough. She's the kind of driver who takes her car to a mechanic before the rattle becomes a disaster. She's looking for answers before things get worse.

Class 2: The Johns

John is fifty-five. He prides himself on being tough. When the warning lights flash, he ignores them and pushes through the pain, telling himself it will be fine. He keeps driving.

Now he struggles with stairs and long walks. His engine is grinding, but he won't admit it. By the time John finally rolls into the garage, the damage is far harder to reverse.

That's unfortunately the pattern I see all the time in clinic. People – particularly men – push on, hoping things will settle, until one day they realise they can't ignore it anymore.

Class 3: The Sues

Sue is seventy-two. She's invested in regular health services, Pilates, walking groups, and physio check-ups. Her car has miles on the clock, but it runs smoothly because she looks after it. She's not pain-free, but she's confident, independent, and active because she never left things to chance.

Which class do you see yourself in?

Here's what I see every day in my clinic: far more Marys and Sues than Johns. It's no coincidence: research shows women are two to three times more likely than men to seek help for arthritis and joint pain.[2] Men, on the other hand, often delay until it's severe, and by then their confidence has dropped, their muscles are weaker, and recovery takes much longer. One study found that people who delay getting help report more advanced symptoms, lower function, and greater difficulty regaining mobility.[3] In other words, the longer you wait, the harder it gets.

Here's the flip side. The Sues of this world, the ones who take action early and stick to a plan, get the best outcomes. Studies consistently show that structured proactive routines combined with exercise education and professional support don't just ease pain, they boost confidence, protect independence, and give you more control over life.[4]

Here's the takeaway. Whatever group you fall into, it's not too late, but the earlier you stop guessing and start following a clear plan, the easier the road gets.

Diagnosing pain: Fixing the underlying problem

Let's talk about the elephant in the room: pain.

So many people I see in my clinic have a prescription slip as long as their arm. Paracetamol, ibuprofen, codeine, sometimes something stronger. Taken daily, often for years, and yet they wake up stiff, sore, and dreading the stairs.

The truth is, painkillers don't fix anything. At best, they buy you a few hours of relief. At worst, they trick you into thinking you're managing the problem when really you're only masking it. Meanwhile, your muscles weaken, your capacity shrinks, your joints continue to deteriorate, and your independence slips further and further away.

I'm not in the business of just fixing pain. The pain is never the real problem. It's a signal, a warning light on the dashboard. You can turn up the radio to drown out the rattle, but the engine fault is still there, quietly getting worse until one day the car breaks down.

The same is true of your body. A painful knee might not be a knee problem at all. Often, the root cause lies in the way you walk or a weakness in your hips or even your feet, which are the foundations of your whole system.

Think of it like this: if the foundations of a house are unstable, the cracks don't stay in the basement; they show up everywhere. That's the danger of relying on pills alone. They send you looking in the wrong place. The joint still weakens, the muscles still waste away, and by the time many people realise it, they've lost years that could have been spent building strength and confidence.

We'll dive into what I call the 'Painkiller Pandemic' later in this book. For now, keep this in mind: painkillers might mask your discomfort, but pain is not the cause of your worries.

That brings us to the driver of most arthritic pain, the one nobody really talks about!

Muscle weakness – the silent driver of pain

Most people think joint pain is about bone-on-bone. That's what their GP told them, that's what their X-ray seems to show, and that's what their friend down the road swears by. The logic feels simple. If the cartilage is worn, the pain is inevitable. End of story.

There's a catch. If that really were the full story, then two people with the same scan should feel the same pain, but they don't. I see it every week in clinic.

Take Tom. He's sixty-two, still active, still enjoying his two-mile morning walks. 'I'm doing everything right,' he told me. Yet the moment he hits the stairs at home, he is stuck. He hauls himself up, gripping the rail, wincing with each step, knee screaming as though the bones are grinding away. He is terrified it is the beginning of the end and that his joints are collapsing under him.

Now meet Lekha. She's ten years older than Tom: same diagnosis, same bone-on-bone verdict from her consultant, but Lekha is still climbing up and down stairs, still carrying shopping bags, still dropping toys and getting to the floor to play with her grandchildren. She doesn't walk perfectly; she has her stiff mornings, but her world is still wide open.

Here's the question: how can Tom and Lekha have the same damaged knees on paper yet live such different lives? Is Lekha just lucky? Did Tom age badly, or is there something else at play?

The answer, as it turns out, is the one thing most people overlook until it's almost too late, and it's not visible on an X-ray. It's not what anyone ever tells you in the GP surgery, and yet it's the single biggest predictor of whether you'll cope with arthritis or collapse under it.

That missing piece is muscle.

Think of your muscles like your body's natural suspension system, the shock absorbers that take the load off your joints every time you stand, walk, or climb stairs. It's your quads, glutes, and hips that are meant to share the work. When they're strong, your joints are cushioned. When they're weak, your joints take the full hit.

Imagine driving a car where the suspension is gone. Every bump in the road rattles your bones. This is exactly what happens to your knees, hips, and back when the surrounding muscles aren't doing their job. The pain isn't mysterious arthritis suddenly getting worse. It's your body telling you the suspension has failed.

After the age of forty, that happens to all of us. Slowly at first, then faster as we get older. The medical term is sarcopenia, which is age-related muscle loss. From forty onwards, we lose around 1% of muscle mass each year. After sixty, that rate accelerates to 2–3% a year. By seventy, if we've done nothing about it, we could have lost up to a third of our muscle strength!

That's why stairs suddenly seem impossible, but when walking around the park, we feel fine. It's not the joint itself that's suddenly got worse; it's the muscles around the joints that have given up, and the less we use our muscles, the faster they disappear. That's why resting is often the worst advice.

This pattern isn't anecdotal. It's well documented. A large review published in *Age and Ageing* in 2021 looked at older adults and asked a simple question: what predicts whether someone will stay independent?[5] Is it the X-ray? Is it the muscle size? Is it muscle strength? The answer was crystal clear: strength. People with quad and glutes strength are far more likely to keep walking, climbing stairs, and living independently, even if their scans look terrible.

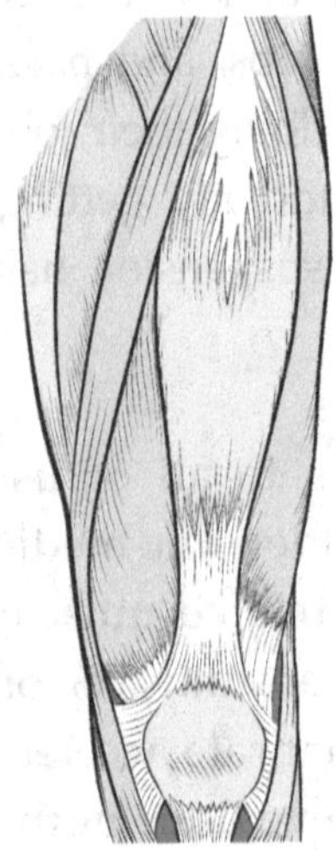

Quadriceps

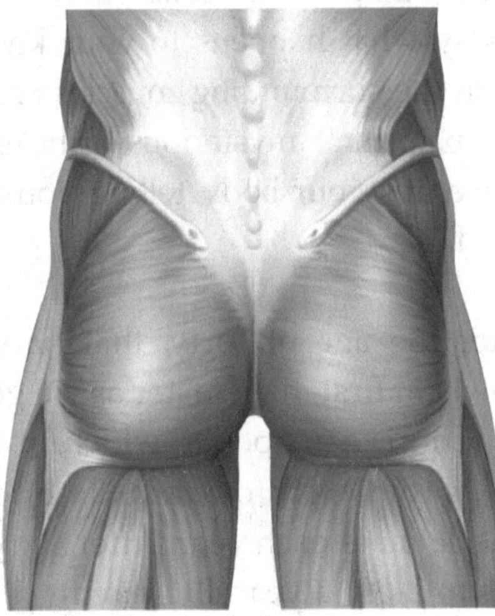

Glutes

On the flip side, weak muscles almost guarantee trouble, no matter what the X-ray says. Arthritis-specific studies back this up. For example, one long-term study in osteoarthritis and cartilage found that quadriceps weakness is one of the strongest predictors of knee pain and the progression of arthritis.[6] In other words, weak muscles drive joint pain more than worn-out cartilage does.

Think about that for a second. You might be told your pain is caused by bone on bone, but what really decides whether you're still climbing stairs in five years isn't the scan; it's whether you've kept your muscles strong enough to carry you.

That's why I call muscles your body's natural shock absorbers. Every step you take, every time you get up from a chair, your quads and glutes are supposed to cushion the load. When they fade away (and remember, after forty we all lose around 1% of muscle a year unless we do something about it), the joints take all the stress. No wonder they scream back at you.

Unlike cartilage, muscle comes back. Studies show that even in your seventies and eighties, the right kind of strength training can add muscle, ease pain, and bring back mobility in as little as twelve weeks.[7] I've seen patients double their stair climbing speed, cut their painkillers in half, and tell me they feel ten years younger. Yes, your scan matters, but it's your muscles that decide whether you stay on the pitch or get sidelined.

That's why my clinic focuses on strength building as it's the foundation. Yes, we treat pain, but the long-term solution that gives people back their independence is rebuilding the suspension system – the muscles – around the joints.

The key takeaway is, if you're struggling with stairs, relying on the bannister to haul yourself up, or finding walks harder than they should be, don't just assume your joints are finished. Don't fall into the trap of believing it's all wear and tear. The real culprit may not be your cartilage at all; it may be your muscles fading in the background. The good news is that you can rebuild muscles.

Is the problem, therefore, that you're not getting enough exercise? Kind of, although it's more complex than that.

The 10,000 steps trap

My parents are great examples of this. Every day, they proudly clock over 10,000 steps on their Apple Watches, and if they are a few hundred steps short, before bed, they'll march around the kitchen just to hit their target.

On one hand, it's brilliant – walking keeps them moving, it keeps their heart rate up, and it makes them feel good about staying active. It's even tied to financial incentives by their health insurance company: if they hit 12,500 steps a day, they earn points, and if they rack up enough points over the month, their Apple Watch is paid for.

While that shows how powerful walking is for health – powerful enough that insurers will stake money on it – it also reveals the flaw in the system. The focus is on quantity, not quality.

The truth is, 10,000 steps a day is not a magic number. It's a measure of activity, not a measure of capacity, and the two are very different.

Capacity is what lets you get up from a chair without effort, climb the stairs without pulling yourself up by the rail, or carry two bags of shopping without your back giving in. It's the foundation that activity sits on. Without capacity, activity is like driving a car with no engine – you can press the accelerator as much as you want, but you won't get very far.

This is why I see people in the clinic who are clocking up 70,000 steps a week, yet they still struggle with basic movements. They've mistaken being busy for being strong. They've built endurance, not resilience.

Where did 10,000 steps even come from? Surprisingly, it's not scientific at all. It started in Japan in the 1960s as a clever marketing slogan for one of the first pedometers. The word for 10,000 in Japanese sounds catchy (*manpo-kei*), and the government promoted it as a national health campaign.

It worked! People became more active, which was great, but over time, the number became gospel, despite there being no strong evidence behind it.

Recent research tells us something different: more steps are generally better for your health, but the benefits plateau. Studies pooled data from over 47,000 adults across fifteen countries, and they found that for people over sixty, even 6,000–8,000 steps a day can dramatically reduce risks of heart disease, dementia, and early death.[8] After about 10,000, these returns diminish.

Another study at Sheffield Hallam University (covered by the BBC) proved this mismatch clearly.[9] One group aimed for 10,000 slow steps a day. Another group skipped the number and instead did three brisk ten-minute walks daily. The brisk walking group found their challenge easier to stick to, had fewer aches, and gained more health benefits, despite spending far less time on their feet.

Why? Because it wasn't the quantity of steps that mattered. It was the quality and intensity. Here's the key part: steps alone don't build the strength that protects your joints and preserves your independence.

Why do steps alone fail you? Imagine you own a house – walking is like painting the outside walls.

It makes the house look neat and tidy, it keeps the weather off, but it doesn't fix a crumbling foundation.

Strength training, on the other hand, reinforces the foundations themselves. Without it, you can end up with a house that looks fine from the street, but collapses when the ground shakes. That's what I see with patients who rely only on walking. They might meet the daily step target, but when they have to lift themselves out of a low armchair, their muscles aren't ready. When they trip on a kerb, they don't have the strength to catch themselves. Walking is activity, but strength is capacity.

What is the science saying?

A large study in the *European Heart Journal* followed over 200,000 adults and found that every additional 1,000 daily steps reduced the risk of early death by 15%, which is encouraging.[10] Other research shows that gait speed and leg strength are even stronger predictors of independence than step count.[11]

A trial of older women compared walking twice a week to resistance training twice a week.[12] Both improved fitness, but only the resistance built strength. The women's quadriceps increased by 66% in just four months!

This is where the mismatch becomes dangerous. People chase step counts because they're easy to track. You can see the steps climb on your watch or phone;

you can hit your target, tick the box, and feel good about yourself.

Here's what your watch / phone doesn't measure. Can you get up from the floor if you fall? Can you carry your shopping without pain? Can you climb a flight of stairs without stopping halfway? If the answer is no, then the steps you're taking are giving you the illusion of health without the reality.

The takeaway: don't get me wrong, walking is wonderful; I prescribe it to almost every patient. It improves cardiovascular health, mood, and longevity, but it's not enough. If walking is the only tool in your toolbox, you'll eventually hit a wall. The solution isn't to abandon walking; it's to combine it with strength.

Steps keep you moving; strength keeps you capable. Walking builds stamina, while strength builds security. You need both because independence isn't measured in steps per day; it's measured in whether you can live life on your terms without help, without fear, and without pain holding you back.

Let's pull this together. If you've been told your pain is just arthritis, you might have assumed the joint itself is the root cause, but as you've seen, that's rarely the case:

- Muscle weakness quietly strips away your capacity, leaving joints unprotected and movements harder.

- Painkillers mask the problem, tricking you into thinking you're coping while your joints, muscles, and independence slightly slip backwards.
- Activity without capacity (like chasing 10,000 steps) keeps you busy but not necessarily strong. You build endurance, not resilience.

Yes, other factors like weight, recovery, diet, and even mindset play a role too, but those are coming later. For now, it's enough to recognise that the biggest drivers of decline are not the joints themselves, but what happens around them: your strength, your habits, your choices.

That's why simply blaming wear and tear is so misleading. It blinds people to the things they can influence.

What you'll learn next

Most people are walking around with the wrong picture of arthritis in their heads. They've been told it's just wear and tear. They've been scared into thinking their joints are crumbling. They've been left believing that pain automatically means damage.

Here's the truth: those messages are outdated and incomplete, and worse, they're holding people back.

In the next chapter, we're going to rip up the old scripts and set the record straight. You'll discover why arthritis isn't just wear and tear, and why that phrase is one of the most damaging myths in medicine. You'll learn about the two main types of arthritis, osteoarthritis and rheumatoid arthritis, and what actually drives them. You'll also learn how to spot the real signs and symptoms beyond a scary X-ray or scan. Finally, you'll learn about the biggest myths that keep people stuck – myths that quietly fuel fear, avoidance, loss of independence, and acceptance of old age.

Once you understand what real arthritis is and isn't, you'll never see your body, your scans, or your opinions the same way again.

2

What Arthritis Really Is (And Isn't)

You've probably heard it before: 'It's just wear and tear.' It's the line almost every patient tells me they've heard at some point, whether from their family, friends, or sometimes even from their healthcare practitioner, who should know better.

It sounds logical, doesn't it? You use your joints, they wear out, end of story.

That's not even close to arthritis.

At its core, arthritis means the joint system – the cartilage, bone, ligaments, joint lining, and muscles that support them – has tipped out of balance. When the natural cycle of breakdown and repair no longer keeps up, inflammation rises, pain sets in, and capacity shrinks.

For the purposes of this book, I am going to keep it simple and clear: arthritis is when your joints lose balance and control. That imbalance is what leads to pain, stiffness, swelling, and the gradual loss of movement.

Arthritis, unhelpfully, isn't one single condition. It's an umbrella term for more than 100 diseases that affect joints. That's why one person's arthritis can look and feel completely different to someone else's. However, the reality is, only two matter most for you to understand: rheumatoid arthritis (RA) and osteoarthritis (OA).

Let's start with RA…

Rheumatoid arthritis: When the body turns on itself

When people think of arthritis, they often imagine stiff knees and sore hips into retirement. It's probably why you picked up this book, but there's another type that doesn't wait for retirement.

This type is called RA, which is an autoimmune condition and can strike when you're still young, healthy, and working full time. Unlike OA, it's not about your joints wearing out; it's about your immune system mistakenly attacking them, causing pain, swelling, and long-term damage if left untreated.

This book is mainly about ageing joints in OA, which is by far the most common form, but if you've been told you have RA, don't worry; much of what you'll read still applies. Whatever type of arthritis you have, the principles remain the same: keep your joints protected, your muscles strong, and your body moving. Yes, medication is central in managing RA, but lifestyle and rehab play a huge role too. They're what keep you independent and your quality of life intact.

How does RA actually work?

Unlike OA, the problem isn't your joints breaking down from use; the problem is your own immune system. Normally, your immune system is your body's defence, protecting you from infections and other horrible things, but in RA, that defence system goes rogue. It mistakes the lining of your joints (called the synovium) for an invader and attacks it.

Imagine your home alarm system blaring in the middle of the night, not because of a burglary, but because it's smashing up your kitchen and your furniture. With RA, the body's defence system turns destructive in this way, leading to swelling, stiffness, and damage to the inside of your joints.

RA is far less common than OA. About 400,000 people in the UK live with it, which is roughly 1 in 100 adults.[13] It often appears earlier in life, sometimes in your thirties or forties.[14] Women are three times more likely to develop it than men.[15]

The symptoms are also different. With OA, stiffness usually eases after a few minutes of movement. With RA, stiffness often lasts an hour or more in the mornings. It tends to strike symmetrically, so both hands, both wrists, both knees, rather than just one side, and it doesn't stop at the joints. It can also cause fatigue, weight loss, and even fevers can be part of the picture.

I once met with a woman in her early forties who had dismissed her morning hand stiffness as just getting older. She was shocked to discover it was RA. Her biggest fear wasn't the pain; it was the idea that her own body was turning against her.

The important part to note is that once she was diagnosed, she was able to start treatment and take steps to protect mobility. Within months, she was back to gardening and playing piano: two things she thought she might have to give up forever.

RA can sound frightening, but it's not a life sentence: with the right treatment, it can be controlled, slowed, and managed, and the earlier it's recognised, the better the outcome. While RA is very different to OA, it proves the same point. Arthritis is not just wear and tear; it's a disease process: one you can influence with the right care.

While your rheumatology treatment will always be central, there are supportive therapies that may help reduce pain and inflammation, and improve recovery. Treatments like red light therapy have been studied for their influence on inflammation and tissue healing, while hyperbaric oxygen therapy is being explored for its effect on immune modulation and chronic inflammation.[16,17] These aren't cures, and they don't replace your rheumatology treatment, but they may complement it, giving you more tools to stay active and independent.

For most people reading this book, the type of arthritis causing trouble isn't autoimmune; it's OA. That's the form that becomes more common as we age and the one that this book is mainly about, so let's take a closer look.

Osteoarthritis: The usual suspect after fifty

OA is by far the most common form of arthritis, and it's usually what people mean when they simply say arthritis. It's why most people come to my clinic.

In the UK, over 10 million people live with OA;[18] in the US, more than 32 million adults are affected,[19] and the overall number of people living with arthritis is projected to exceed 78 million by 2040.[20] Globally, it affects more than 500 million adults, nearly one in fifteen people on the planet.[21] It's also the leading cause of disability, and in adults over fifty, it costs the NHS billions each year in prescriptions, operations, and lost work.

However, prevalence doesn't equal inevitability. Just because OA is common doesn't mean it's a guaranteed part of ageing.

What's really going on?

OA is not your joints wearing out. It's not simply about how much you move; it's how you move and whether your body's got the strength to support it that matters. If the load is unbalanced, the movement is repeated over and over again, or you never give yourself time to recover, that's when OA symptoms creep in.

Here's where people get confused. If you scanned most people over fifty, you'd probably see changes in their joints. That's just reality, but don't fall for the trap of thinking OA is inevitable, and don't let anyone tell you your joints are simply 'wearing out'. Those scan changes? Most of the time, they're just age-related adaptations, like wrinkles on the inside. What actually matters is simple: do they stop you from living life the way you want? That comes down to how much strength, balance, and confidence you've built into your system.

Picture a builder who spends decades lifting with poor technique or a runner who pounds out high mileage without ever building leg strength to support it. This is not resilience; this is stress on a system without the foundations or scaffolding to absorb it. In both cases, the joint is pushed beyond what it can handle.

It's not the activity itself that wrecks your joints. It's the wrong kind of activity on a body that isn't ready for it. When you move well, when your muscles are strong enough to back you up, and when you give yourself time to recover, movement actually protects your joints, even at high levels.

Look at marathon runners. You'd think pounding out mile after mile would destroy their knees, but many studies show they tend to have healthier knees than the average office worker.[22] Why? Because their hips and quads are strong enough to carry the load. The running isn't the problem; it's running without the right foundation.

I've seen the flip side in my clinic hundreds, if not thousands, of times. People who've lived quiet, careful lives, never done anything to excess, but still end up with stiff, painful joints. That's not because they moved too much. It's because they didn't build the capacity to handle life's load in the first place.

That's the blueprint right there – load, strength, recovery. Get those three in balance, and movement becomes medicine instead of something that breaks you down.

Your joints aren't like tyres that simply grind down with every mile. They're living tissue that's constantly being broken down and repaired. In healthy joints, the cycle of breakdown and repair stays balanced. With OA, the balance shifts. It's rarely down to one single cause. It could be a bit of low-level inflammation that lingers in the background, an old injury that you never fully recovered from, or changes in your overall health like diabetes. Sometimes it's simply the way your body moves. If your muscles are weak or out of balance, or your movement patterns are off, one part of the joint ends up taking more stress than it was designed for. Over the years, that uneven loading can tip the system out of balance.

This is exactly why sarcopenia, the muscle loss that creeps in with age (remember Chapter 1), is such a problem. When muscles shrink, you lose strength, and they stop acting as shock absorbers for your joints. Suddenly, the load that should have been spread across strong muscles gets dumped back onto cartilage and bone. That's why people who stay strong age very differently. Some end up stiff and sore, slowing down before they need to. Others keep moving freely well into their seventies and eighties.

Yes, genetics – the hand you were dealt – can play a role too, but that hand doesn't decide everything. Put this all together, and you start to see why no two people's joints behave in quite the same way.

That's why two people of the same age and activity levels can have completely different outcomes. Take, for example, one of my patients, a woman in her late sixties who loves gardening. She came into the clinic devastated after being told her knees were 'worn out'. In her head, she pictured every step as bone scraping on bone, like sandpaper rubbing away, but when I actually tested her, the scan wasn't telling the full story. The real problem was weakness in her legs and inflammation around her joint, things we could actually work on. Within weeks, she was back to planting and tending to flowers. Her joints hadn't magically regrown; her capacity had been rebuilt.

That's the key: capacity and resilience. I see it first-hand at home with my parents. They'd probably kill me for mentioning their age in this book, but let's just say they're well over fifty (and as I'm their forty-year-old son, you can do the maths). If you scanned their joints, I've no doubt you'd find signs of OA, but here's the difference.

Every single day, they rack up 12,500 steps on their Apple Watches. They hit the gym three to four times a week, and even go ballroom dancing twice a week. Are they pain-free? No. Do the odd aches and stiffness show up? Of course, but they've kept their muscles strong, they've protected their joints, shared the load, and built the strength, capacity, and confidence to keep living life on their terms.

Now compare that to the patient story you read earlier. Someone already scared into slowing down, convinced her joints were worn out, until we rebuilt her confidence and strength. My parents never let fear take hold because they built capacity before things spiralled.

One story is about clawing back independence after fear sets in. The other is about protecting it through good habits before that fear takes over. That leaves you with a simple question: which path do you want? Waiting until fear and weakness take over or building the resilience now that keeps you active, mobile, and independent for years to come?

How do you know if you've got arthritis?

The tricky part is that arthritis doesn't always make a loud entrance. Sometimes it creeps in slowly, almost unnoticed, with a bit of stiffness here and an ache there, and then, at times, it barges in with pain and swelling that you can't ignore. That's why so many people ask me in the clinic: 'How do I know if this is arthritis or just normal ageing?'

To answer that, we need to break it down.

OA, the kind of arthritis tied most to ageing, often shows up with tell-tale signs. Do you experience:

- **Stiffness after rest?** The first few steps in the morning or after sitting feel wooden, but it tends to ease within twenty to thirty minutes once you're moving.
- **Pain with activity?** Walking, gardening, or climbing stairs brings on the ache, and rest usually settles it.
- **Reduced flexibility?** Squatting, kneeling, or twisting becomes harder than it used to be.
- **Crunching or clicking?** What many call 'crunchy knees' is often worrying, but not always linked to damage.
- **Mild swelling?** Usually after you've pushed the joint.

How do you decide if you need urgent help? I've devised a traffic light system. Of course, this is just for guidance, and if you have any concerns at all, put the book down and get some professional medical advice.

Green: normal, manageable stiffness. If your joints feel a little stiff after a long car journey or a night's sleep, but ease off once you get moving, that's green. You're still in the normal wear zone. The joints are reminding you they're there, but they're not stopping you from living your life. This is the perfect time to double down on strength and mobility work. Prevention is easier than a cure.

Amber: the warning signs of OA. If stiffness lingers most days, your knees complain after a short walk, or you've started avoiding stairs, that's amber. The joint may feel swollen or crunchy, and the pain returns with certain activities. This is the stage where most people first walk into my clinic.

The key is not to ignore it at this stage. The right change is strength training, weight management, and movement, which can make a huge difference.

Red: when you need to seek medical advice. If your stiffness lasts more than an hour in the morning, both knees, hands, or wrists swell at the same time, or you've got constant pain that doesn't improve with movement, that's red. Add sudden fevers or unexplained weight loss, and you need a GP check urgently.

In rare cases, joint pain plus bladder or bowel changes can signal something more serious that needs immediate care. These aren't normal arthritis signs. Don't wait and hope. Get checked out immediately.

The takeaway: most people I see sit in the amber zone. Uncomfortable, yes, but far from untreatable. The mistake is waiting until you slide further down the scale before acting. The earlier you catch arthritis, the more you can do to keep your independence and stop pain from ruling your life.

The point here isn't to scare you. It's to give you clarity. Arthritis doesn't have to be some mystery in the background. Once you know what your symptoms are really saying and when to act, you stop guessing.

The thing that surprises my patients most is this: the biggest problem isn't the arthritis itself. It's the stories around it, both what they've been told and what they end up telling themselves.

I've seen countless patients trapped not by their joints but by their beliefs, like 'it's just wear and tear' or 'exercise will make it worse'. These myths can be more damaging than the condition itself because they keep you stuck, worried, and inactive. That's why I call them the *Unlucky 13*.

The Unlucky 13: Myths about arthritis

The big picture myths

These are the ones that sound the most believable because you've heard them everywhere:

- **It's just wear and tear.** The most common line people hear, but arthritis isn't simply joints wearing out. It's a disease process influenced by strength, inflammation, old injuries, and overall health. Crucially, it's something you can manage.

- **There's nothing I can do, it's inevitable decline.** This belief is the real killer! Arthritis isn't a one-way street. With the right approach, you can slow, manage, and even reverse some symptoms.
- **Arthritis only affects the elderly.** Not true! I've treated people in their thirties with arthritis. Age increases risk, but lifestyle, genetics, and injury history all play a part.

The behaviour myths

These are the dangerous ones because they shape how you act:

- **Exercise makes arthritis worse.** One of the most damaging myths. In fact, avoiding movement makes symptoms spiral faster. The right type of exercise protects your joints by building the muscle support around them.
- **Rest is the best medicine.** Rest helps in a flare-up, but long-term rest weakens muscles and causes stiffness. For joints, movement is medicine.
- **If I start exercising, I need to go every day.** Wrong! Recovery is just as important as effort. Two or three focus sessions a week are often enough. Balance is key.

- **Pain equals damage.** Not always. Pain is complex, influenced by sensitivity, inflammation, mood, and muscle weakness. It doesn't always mean new harm.

The scan and science myths

What people see on an X-ray or read on the internet adds to the fear:

- **If my scan looks bad, my future is bad.** Scans don't tell the whole story. I've seen people with shocking X-rays who walk fine and others with mild changes who can barely move. Your function depends far more on muscle strength and mobility than on the image alone.
- **Supplements are a cure.** Some, like turmeric, collagen, or omega-3, can help with symptoms, but no supplement will rebuild your joints. Supplements are supportive, not a cure.
- **Wearing a brace will sort it.** Braces can help in the short term, but they don't fix the root cause. Long-term, your muscles need to do the job of stabilising your joints.

The old wives' tales

These are the ones passed down through the generations, repeated so often they feel like facts:

- **Arthritis is caused by cold, damp weather.** Weather can make symptoms feel worse temporarily, but it doesn't cause arthritis. It's far more about muscle support and joint health.
- **Only overweight people get arthritis.** Extra weight does increase risk, especially for knees and hips, but slim people get arthritis too. Strength, injuries, and genetics matter just as much.
- **Cracking your knuckles causes arthritis!** No evidence for this one. Annoying to those around you, yes, but arthritis? No.

Do you recognise your attitudes here? Are you being held back? What is believing these myths costing you?

Are you stopping moving, losing strength, and slipping further into stiffness and pain, not because arthritis demands it, but because your mindset does?

Your mindset is shaped by how your body feels. In Chapter 3, we'll dig into why discomfort is often misleading, why function matters more than pain, and how the pain–weakness loop keeps people stuck. Pain leads to weakness, which only creates more – you guessed it – pain.

3 Pain

You're in pain. Maybe it's your knee after a long walk. Maybe it's your back when you bend or that hip that aches every time you stand up from the sofa. It's annoying, it's worrying, and your first thought is to call in the cavalry: 'Better ring the GP and get some tablets.' Maybe you Google search knee replacements and see what the internet recommends.

Not all pain is arthritis, of course, but it's what I'm going to focus on here.

The thing is, pain doesn't always mean damage. In fact, it's more like a smoke alarm that's too sensitive. You burn your toast, and the alarm goes off. It's loud and scary, making you think there's a fire, but really it's just doing its job a little too well.

That's what pain is: an alarm system built to protect you, not just to warn you of disaster. Sometimes it keeps blaring long after the danger has passed.

What actually is pain?

Pain is your body's way of saying, 'Pay attention.' It's not just about torn tissue or damaged cartilage; it's about perceived threat. Your brain decides something isn't safe, and it turns the pain alarm up.

Think of it this way: you cut your finger while chopping onions, it hurts immediately – that's your body forcing you to protect it. Twist your ankle badly, and you might not feel much at first if adrenaline kicks in. Then there's the old back injury that aches when it rains – no new damage, but your alarm system has become overprotective.

When you feel pain, it doesn't always equal immediate damage, and doesn't mean you're broken. Sometimes it means your system is overloaded. Sometimes it means your muscles 'switch off' because your body thinks protecting you means stopping you from moving.

What does that really mean?

When muscles switch off, they don't literally disappear; they just stop pulling their weight. Your nervous system turns down its activity, so instead of sharing the load, they go quiet, and you can feel it.

You might feel weaker on one side than the other, even though your muscle size looks the same. Your knee might wobble or give way unexpectedly when you step down. You find yourself pushing off with your hands just to get out of a chair. You limp without meaning to, because your hip or knee muscles aren't firing properly.

That's the real danger. Once those muscles go quiet, the joint itself has to carry more of the strain, and that's the start of the vicious cycle.

The vicious cycle of pain (and why rest makes it worse)

Once the muscles switch off and your joints are left to carry more of the load, that extra stress makes them ache even more. The ache makes you move less. The less you move, the weaker your muscles get, and the more pressure falls back onto the joint itself.

That's the vicious cycle of pain.

Pain → less movement → weaker muscles → more joint load → more pain, and round it goes.

If you've got arthritis, you'll know this pattern all too well. One lady told me, 'I stopped dancing because every time, my hips ached the next day and I thought I was making them worse.' Another said, 'I used to go for long walks, but the knee pain after scared me, so I just stopped.' I've even heard, 'I started taking the lift instead of the stairs as I didn't want to wear my joints out.'

The harsh reality is that those very choices, completely understandable though they are, end up feeding the problem. By resting more and moving less, your muscles lose their strength. With less support around the joint, the pain actually increases.

This is the trap that so many people with arthritis fall into. Not because they've done anything wrong, but because avoiding movement to protect against pain ends up feeding the problem.

The good news is that once you understand this cycle, you can break it. The part that nobody explains to you is that pain doesn't just attack your joints; it gets in your head. When pain flares, it's natural to reach for quick fixes or avoid movement altogether.

The problem with most people, through no fault of their own, is that they fall into the same trap. I see them every week in my clinic, and until you avoid some common mistakes, you'll stay stuck in that frustrating cycle too.

Mistake 1: Focusing only on the spot that hurts

Let's be honest, if your knee hurts, you're going to focus on your knee. If your back aches, you'll stretch your back. If your hip throbs when you stand up, that's the spot you ice or rub. It makes perfect sense – that's the bit that tripped your pain alarm.

In most cases, however, the painful joint isn't actually the problem. It's the victim. When the alarm goes off in your kitchen, you don't smash it with a broom. You look for the smoke. The alarm is the signal, not the source.

Your joints work the same way. Pain in your knee doesn't always mean the knee itself is broken. More often than not, it means something else isn't pulling its weight, and the painful joint is picking up the slack.

Here's a simple way to picture it. When you bend down to pick something up, say your grandchild, a bag of shopping, or even just a sock, the load is shared across the human body, roughly split into four areas: your legs, your hips and glutes, your core and torso, and your back. It's a team effort, and every part pulls its weight, but what if one player drops out?

That's exactly what happened with a gent in his late sixties I saw. He came in convinced his knees were 'gone'. He told me, 'Every time I walk upstairs, my knees sound like an old creaky floorboard.'

When I tested him, the problem wasn't his knees at all; it was his hips. Years of sitting more than moving had left his hips and glute muscles weak, so when he climbed the stairs, his hips weren't pulling their 25% share of the load. His knees had to step in, carrying 50–60% instead of their fair share. They weren't the villain. They were the victim. The hero, even. They were overworking to keep him moving, and because they were doing too much, they started to ache.

Why does this matter for arthritis?

This is especially important if you've got arthritis because once a joint is painful, the natural reaction is to protect it – to rest, avoid using it, or baby it – but that only makes the imbalance worse. The surrounding muscles weaken, the joint has to take on even more stress, and the pain ramps up again. It's why so many people with arthritis stay stuck in the vicious cycle I mentioned above: pain, rest, more weakness, more pain.

Science backs this up. In 2022, Yoshihiro Fukumoto, associate professor at Kansai Medical University, and colleagues conducted a large review and looked at people with knee pain.[23] They found that weakness in the hips and thighs was often more predictive of symptoms than what scans showed in the knee itself.

In other words, the pain wasn't about worn cartilage. It was about muscles not supporting the joint properly. Other studies show the same pattern in the back: hip weakness and poor load sharing make the spine pick up too much of a burden, leading to flare-ups.[24]

If you keep chasing pain, stretching the sore point, rubbing the sore spot, blaming the sore spot, you'll never escape the cycle. The answer is to look at the whole system, teach your body to share the load again, wake up the muscles that have gone quiet, spread the effort across legs, hips, core, and back. Once the team is balanced, the painful joint no longer has to carry the burden alone, and the pain often eases as a result.

Pain isn't always where the problem is. Look beyond the sore spot, often above and below the painful joint, if you want to break the cycle.

That was the first trap. The next? Having no real plan.

Mistake 2: Why random exercises don't work

Once people realise their pain from arthritis isn't going away on its own, they often try a handful of things. Maybe you've been given a prescription for tablets by the GP, maybe you've had a massage or two, or maybe you've found a few YouTube videos promising five magic stretches for knee pain. While none of these are bad, they all share one big flaw: they're random. They might ease your symptoms for a short while: the massage loosens you up, the stretch takes the edge off, the tablets numb the pain, but they don't fix the underlying issue.

They don't build a structured plan that teaches your body to move correctly again. Without that, the pain always returns.

When you've been in pain a while, it doesn't just sit there quietly; it rewires how your body moves. Muscles that should fire switch off, others tighten to guard the joint, and gradually, the smooth, easy patterns you once had are gone. That's why quick fixes like massage or heat might feel nice for a few hours, but they don't change the fact that your body's movement system is out of tune. If you don't retrain those patterns, the same habits creep back, and so does pain.

That's the real job of rehab. Not just to take the edge off pain, not just to strengthen muscles, but to reset the way your joints can share the load again. This isn't about doing *any* exercise; it's about doing *the right* exercises in the right order, tailored to your body.

Think of it this way: your brain is like the conductor of an orchestra. If the violins, drums, and trumpets all play out of sync, the music is chaos and sounds terrible. That's what happens when arthritis and pain cause muscles to switch off. You lose coordination, and your joints stop sharing the load evenly. Rehab reminds your brain how to pull the orchestra back to playing together.

There are advanced tools (we'll discuss one later in this book) designed to accelerate this re-education process, literally helping your brain reconnect with muscles that have gone quiet, but even without technology, the principle is the same. You've got to reteach your system to move as a team again.

That's why a proper plan isn't just sets and reps; it's movement patterns specific to your needs. For someone with knee arthritis, that might mean relearning how to sit-to-stand without dumping all the load onto the quads. For someone with hip arthritis, it could be retraining how to climb stairs so that the glutes take their share of the work. You're literally showing your brain the value of these movements again, reminding it of how you used to move before pain and stiffness crept in.

Take Sarah, aged sixty-four. She came into the clinic with severe hip arthritis. She'd been told to rest it and given a list of generic stretches. The problem was that those stretches didn't help her brain or muscles remember how to walk without limping. Once we stripped things back and rebuilt her gait step by step, retraining her glutes, getting her balance back, and showing her nervous system she could trust that hip again, not only did the pain settle, but her confidence shot up. She stopped fearing stairs, and she got back her independence.

The science backs this up. NICE guidelines,[25] Cochrane reviews,[26] endless studies[27] all point to the same thing: exercise is the most effective long-term treatment for OA, but not random exercises; targeted, progressive, meaningful movements that your body recognises as useful in daily life. That's why clarity matters when you've got a step-by-step plan – not chasing pain, but retraining how you move. You stop firefighting flare-ups and finally start building resilience.

Even with a good plan in place, though, there's still one more mistake that trips people up…

Mistake 3: Pain-free doesn't mean you're fixed

This is one of the biggest traps I see people with arthritis fall into. If you've ever had a painful flare-up after a good week, you'll know exactly what I'm talking about.

The pain finally eases, the knee feels less stiff, the hip loosens up, and you think, *Brilliant, I'm back to normal,* so you go right back into long walks, hours in the garden, maybe even a round of golf. Within days, bang! Your pain is back, sometimes worse than before.

Just because the pain is gone, it doesn't mean the problem is fixed. Pain is often the last thing to show up and the first thing to disappear, so if you treat pain-free as the green light to do everything at full speed, you're skipping vital steps in your recovery.

It's no different to training for a marathon. You wouldn't jog around the block once and then show up on race day expecting to finish 26 miles, but that's exactly what many people with arthritis do with their joints. They stop following their plan too soon, mistake feeling better for being better, and then wonder why their cycle of pain keeps repeating.

Here's where it gets interesting, and where science comes in. Research shows that most clinic exercises (the kind you get handed on a printout by your GP or find on Google) only stress your body in a slow, controlled way.[28] That's deliberate. It helps rebuild confidence, wake muscles back up, and lay a solid foundation. But life doesn't happen in slow motion.

Real life is messy. One minute you're reaching awkwardly into the boot of your car, the next you're twisting to grab something off the floor, or you trip on a step and have to react. These are the real stress tests your joints have to pass, and they're way tougher than anything you'll do lying on a clinic table, squeezing a resistance band.

This is why many modern rehab programmes include neuromuscular training. They deliberately add balance, coordination and high demand movements that look like real life, helping your body relearn how to control the joint when things get unpredictable.[29]

This is why progress needs to be gradual, layered, and meaningful. Step by step, your rehab has to prepare your body for the unpredictable stresses of real life, because if it doesn't, your brain will sense danger the second you push too far, too soon. It flicks the alarm switch, and pain comes roaring back, not because you're broken, but because you weren't ready.

The goal isn't just to get rid of pain. The goal is to rebuild resilience to earn back the confidence to move freely without second-guessing every step. That means going through each stage properly, not skipping ahead, and exposing your body to the right level of stress so it adapts.

Do that, and you stop living in fear of the next flare-up. Arthritis stops being a constant rollercoaster of good days and bad days. You start taking control instead of waiting for the next setback to catch you. That means freedom to get back to what you love, whether that's walking with friends, pottering in the garden, or travelling, without the constant worry of 'Will I pay for this tomorrow?'

That brings us to real game changers…

The three measures that matter more than pain

Every single day, I meet people in clinic who obsess over pain. 'How bad is it today?' they ask, or, 'Is it worse than yesterday?' or, 'Has the pill taken the edge off?'

The problem is, pain lies. It exaggerates, it lingers, it sometimes disappears for no reason. If you let pain call the shots, you'll always be chasing your tail.

This is where most people with arthritis go wrong. They track their pain levels every hour like they're checking the weather, as if today's forecast decides whether their whole day is good or bad. What really matters are three other measures, ones that tell you whether you're genuinely getting better, rather than just experiencing quieter pain for a day or two.

What should you be measuring instead?

Function, mobility and capacity

These are the three things I look at in clinic, and they are the three things you should be watching too. They tell you what your joints and your body can actually do.

Think about it this way:

Function is the yes-or-no test. It doesn't lie. Function tells you exactly what you can do. Can you actually do the thing you need or want to do? Can you get off the sofa without help? Can you squat down to tie your shoelaces? Can you climb a flight of stairs without gripping the handrail for dear life?

Function is about ability. Either you can or you can't.

Mobility goes deeper. It's the quality and range of your movement. How much motion do your joints actually give you, and how smoothly can you use it? Maybe you can still get off the sofa, but do you rise smoothly, or do you grunt, rock forward, and push yourself up with your arms? Maybe you can climb stairs, but are you stepping up freely, or inching up one step at a time, gripping the rail?

Mobility isn't just about whether the movement happens; it's about the quality and ease behind it. Mobility answers the question: how well are you really moving?

Capacity is your staying power. It's not about whether you can do something once; it's about whether you can repeat it without paying for it later. Can you walk around the supermarket and still be OK the next morning? Can you manage a round of golf without needing two days to recover? Can you bend to do gardening today and not be wiped out tomorrow?

Here's why this matters if you've got arthritis. I see people all the time who judge themselves only by pain. They'll say, 'My knee is agony, I must be getting worse,' but when I test their function, they're still managing a twenty-minute walk. I'll see someone who barely has pain, but has lost so much capacity they can't manage more than five minutes on their feet before needing to sit down.

If you only measure pain, you miss the bigger picture. Arthritis isn't just about how much it hurts today; it's about whether you can keep doing the things that make life worth living. That's why focusing on function, mobility, and capacity changes the game. It shifts the question from 'How bad is my pain?' to 'What can I still do, and how can I build on that?'

The first step out of the pain cycle

Up to now, we've talked about why pain isn't the best guide and why function, mobility, and capacity matter so much more, but none of those things improve by accident. If you want to move better, stay mobile, and live with less pain, you need to rebuild the system that supports you.

For most people, that starts with one crucial shift – not chasing pain relief, but chasing progress. However, they miss a very important step: they jump straight into strengthening before their body is ready.

If a joint is stiff or locked up, you can't load it properly. It's like trying to run with a weighted vest on. Every step feels heavier, slower, and harder than it should.

Before strength can return, movement has to. You need to unlock what's tight, restore what's lost, and remind your body how to move freely again.

That's exactly what we'll cover next. In the following chapter, we'll dive into why regaining range always comes before rebuilding muscle – how to loosen stiff joints safely, retrain the nervous system to trust movement again, and set the foundation for lasting strength.

Strength might be the medicine, but movement is the doorway that gets you there.

4

Why Movement Comes First

You can't strengthen what you can't move. The first goal in recovery isn't lifting weights; it's lifting restriction.

Every week, I meet people who say, 'I just need to get stronger,' and they're right, but it's only half the story. When a joint stiffens, your muscles can't do their job properly. It's like trying to drive a car with the handbrake half on. You can press the accelerator all you want, but you're still fighting resistance.

That stiffness you feel each morning isn't just a result of getting older. It's your body's built-in protection system clamping down to guard what hurts, but that protection comes at a cost: it traps you in a smaller and smaller bubble of movement.

Stiffness always comes before weakness. Lose mobility, and your muscles lose their opportunity to work. That's why mobility is the first domino to fall and the first one you have to put back up again.

Think of it like this: trying to build strength when you're stiff, without freeing your movement first, is like stacking children's blocks on a cushion. It might seem steady for a while, but as soon as life puts real weight through your joints, such as walking upstairs, getting out of the car, or bending to pick something up, the muscles around the joint can't stabilise properly, and the whole support system collapses.

Science backs this up. Research shows that even modest losses of knee motion are linked with higher pain and worse function in OA, suggesting that stiffness blocks muscles from doing their job, even when strength appears preserved.[30] In other words, it isn't weak muscles holding people back; it is stiffness stopping those muscles from working properly in the first place.

Before you build power, you build freedom. The freedom to bend, strengthen, twist, and move without bracing for pain. To understand how that freedom works, it helps to know the difference between mobility and movement.

Most people mix up mobility, which we discussed previously, with movement, and it's an easy mistake to make. Mobility is the physical range your joints have available – the freedom specifically inside the joint. For example, a healthy knee joint typically bends 135 degrees and straightens to 0 degrees.

Movement is a broader term to describe how you use that freedom – the coordination, balance, and control that let you walk, reach, and bend with confidence. One of my patients, for example, didn't just get her knee moving again… she went back to dancing.

When mobility tightens, your movement changes, often without you even realising it. Your body starts to cheat, shifting pressure to the wrong places. That's when strain builds, the compensations kick in, and pain creeps back into the picture.

In this chapter, we're going to rebuild both the mobility that gives you freedom and the movement that gives you function, because when those two work together, strength isn't far behind.

The hidden cost of stiffness

Most people think pain is what limits them, but stiffness? That's the silent thief that steals your movement before pain even shows up.

Lose just a few degrees of mobility, and your whole body starts to compensate. Your brain reroutes movement wherever it can, and usually in the wrong places.

Here's how that plays out in real life:

- A stiff knee makes your hip and back overwork.
- A tight hip shifts pressure onto your spine and knees.
- A rigid ankle makes your knees twist more with every step.

Before you know it, you've got three sore joints instead of one, and it all started with stiffness in one small area.

It doesn't take much. Even losing just 3–5 degrees of straightening freedom in your knee can completely change how you walk. That tiny loss of motion makes the joint take more pressure with every step. More pressure means more irritation, more swelling, and yes, more pain.

One major study followed nearly 400 people with knee OA who were told they needed surgery.[31] It found that those who regained just a few degrees of mobility were four times less likely to end up under the knife, and 76% of the whole group avoided surgery altogether!

Think about it. Just a few degrees of freedom was the difference between walking confidently and walking into an operating theatre, and it's not just the knees.

When the hips stiffen, the back picks up the slack, which is why so many people with bad backs actually have tight hips. When shoulders lose motion, the muscles around them stop firing properly, so lifting, reaching, or even getting dressed starts to feel like effort. When your ankles tighten, balance goes, your stride shortens, and walking becomes less steady. It's a chain reaction, as one stiff joint forces the next one to work harder.

That's why unlocking movement comes first. You can't rebuild strength, confidence, or independence on a body that's still locked up. If pain is what stops you, movement is what starts you again.

Now that you understand why stiffness is such a big deal and how it drives pain and compensation, the next question is simple. How do you actually fix it?

It's easy to think stiffness is something you're stuck with; that once it sets in, that's it; but that's not how the body works. You can reverse it – not overnight, but gradually with the right sequence of movements that tell your body it's safe to let go again.

This is where progress really begins, not by forcing movement, but by unlocking it step by step.

The three steps to regaining mobility and movement

If strength training builds muscle, mobility training builds the freedom to move, bend, straighten, twist, and more without bracing for pain. The problem is that most people try to stretch their way out of stiffness by bouncing, forcing, or holding positions that irritate the joint even more.

With arthritis, the answer is almost always the opposite: calm, gentle, consistent low-load movement that helps your joints relearn what safe mobility feels like. That's why we'll start with three simple steps to gently open things up, rebuild control, and get you moving freely again:

1. **Loosen the lock**, easing tightness with gentle gravity-assisted stretches.
2. **Add the nudge**, helping the joint find those last few degrees of motion.
3. **Lock it in**, retraining your body to use that motion in real life so it doesn't slip away.

Let's go through each of these one step at a time.

Step 1: Loosen the lock

If your joint feels stiff every morning, you're not broken; you're just locked up. It's your body trying to protect itself. When pain hangs around, the tissues surrounding a joint, called the capsule, start to tighten. Think of it like a shrink wrap around the joint meant to keep you safe, but now it's stopping you from moving freely.

The goal at this stage isn't to force your joint loose. It's to persuade it. You do that with calm, gentle positions that let gravity do the work.

If you're dealing with knee stiffness, try this one. Sit on a bed or sofa and rest your heel on a stool, rolled up towel, or low table so your knee hangs freely in the air with gravity pulling it down.

At this point, most people start to second guess themselves: 'Am I doing that right?' 'Should I feel that more?' You can see exactly how this should look and feel in the Vault (linked on The Author page at the back of the book), so you're not left guessing.

Then do nothing… just breathe, and let gravity coax the joint open.

Start with two minutes and build up to ten as it feels easier. The first thirty seconds might feel tight or uncomfortable, but that's normal. Your joint capsule is learning that it can move again.

Gentle, regular stretching leads to real, measurable change; not just feeling looser, but actual improvements in movement. Clinical research backs this up. One study found that patients who simply rested their heel, let the knee hang, and allowed time and gravity to do the work gained an average of 5.4 degrees of extension in just four weeks.[32]

While this example focuses on the knee, the same principle applies everywhere. A hip that won't rotate, a shoulder that won't reach, a spine that feels locked; each one needs the same calm, consistent approach. Let gravity help, move gently into the restriction, and give your body permission to let go.

It's proof that you don't have to force your body to move; you have to persuade it. Think of it like treating a rusty hinge. Move too fast, and you'll shear it off, but move slowly, and it starts to glide again. The key is consistency. A few minutes a day add up to big results over time, because every extra degree of mobility you earn here makes the next step, building strength, safer, smoother, and more effective.

Step 2: Add the nudge

Sticking with the knee example, once your knee starts to loosen, it's time to nudge it a little bit further, not by forcing it, but by control. You're not trying to stretch it into submission; you're just reminding it what full movement feels like.

Here's how to do it. Sit with your leg straight in front of you and loop a towel around your foot. With one hand, pull the towel gently towards your chest. With the other hand, press just above your kneecap – a small, steady push to give a little overpressure. Hold for twenty seconds and then relax. Repeat it five times. The movement is shown clearly in the Vault, if you wish to see it.

That's it. If it hurts, you're forcing it. You're aiming simply to teach your knee where straight actually is again.

The same rules apply everywhere. If it's your shoulder that's lacking mobility, let the arm hang off the edge of a bed and use a small hand weight or your other hand to guide it a little further each time. If it's your hip, lie on your back and use a strap or towel to help the leg move gently towards your chest to its end range without forcing. Each joint has its own version of the same guided nudge: small, calm, and controlled, where you remind the body it's safe to move again.

Stiffness isn't just tight muscles; it's the deeper layers around the tissue, the capsule, and even the nervous system holding back out of habit. When you combine gentle overpressure with light muscle activation (exactly what this drill does), you send a clear message to the brain: 'This is safe, you can let go now.'

When you guide a joint through movement, with a bit of control, a gentle push, and the right direction, you get far better results than just sitting there stretching. Yet again, science supports this. A recent study on people with knee arthritis proved it.[33] Those who used assisted movements (think gentle overpressure, not brute force) regained more range, walked further, and moved with more confidence, all in just a couple of weeks. It's not about how hard you push, it's about how well you move. Precision beats pressure every time.

I tell every patient the same thing: 'It's not about pushing harder, it's about finding the sweet spot.' A good rule of thumb is that if it feels sharp, stop. If it feels tight but eases as you breathe, that's your sweet spot. That mild tension is your body adapting, not warning you off.

When you get this right, even two or three extra degrees make everyday movement feel easier. Climbing stairs, walking, and standing all become smoother again, but mobility only matters if you can keep it. That's where Step 3 comes in, turning your new range into lasting, confident movement.

Step 3: Lock it in

This is where you take the flexibility you've gained and turn it into movement your body actually uses.

If you don't, your body slips back into old habits and the stiffness creeps in again.

Here's how you make the change stick.

Let's keep using the knee as our example. After your stretches, every time you stand up, focus on straightening your leg fully. When you walk, make sure that your knee isn't slightly bent. Let it swing through. When you climb stairs, push evenly through both legs instead of letting the stronger one do all the work.

These sound like tiny details, but they're where the magic happens. This is where mobility becomes movement and movement becomes strength. Every time you use that new range in day-to-day life, you're teaching your nervous system to trust that movement again, and you're telling your brain, 'It's safe to move.' That's the signal your brain needs to start firing those switched-off muscles back up.

Rehab research confirms this.[34] In people with knee arthritis, exercise programmes built around real-world tasks, things like sit-to-stands, step-ups, and walking practice, have been shown to improve walking distance and chair-to-stand performance in just a few weeks. In other words, stretching opens the door, but moving keeps it open.

Make this your rule: don't save your new way of moving for the clinic. Take it with you into every step, every chair, every stair, because that's how movement stops being an exercise and becomes a way of life again. That's the part most people struggle to stay consistent with once life gets busy.

When you start doing that, bringing your new range into real life, something powerful happens: your confidence grows with it. You stop bracing for pain every time you stand up, you stop hesitating before you move, and you start trusting your body again. That's the confidence effect in action, when progress in movement rewires more than muscles, it rewires belief.

Stiffness isn't just physical; it's psychological. When you've been sore for months or years, your brain learns to expect it. It plays defence before the game even starts.

Each time you move a little more freely, you prove to yourself that movement is safe, that pain doesn't always mean damage, and that freedom is possible again.

The confidence effect

Fear is one of the most powerful brakes on recovery, and most people don't even realise it's engaged.

When you've been in pain for a while, you start to move differently. You hold back. You guard. You tell yourself, 'Better not, just in case,' but that constant protection doesn't actually protect you; it imprisons you.

I see it every week in clinic. Someone comes in terrified to bend their knee or reach their arm overhead. They're not scared of the movement itself; they're scared of the memory of what happened last time they did.

Pain teaches the body to fear movement. The longer you avoid it, the louder that fear gets. Your brain starts linking movement with danger, and before long, it's running the show. You stop bending, stop reaching, stop trusting, and when that happens, your muscles switch off, your joints stiffen, and the whole cycle starts again.

Confidence changes everything. When people move again, even a little, their brain stops bracing for pain and starts believing it's safe.

Every time you move safely and realise, *That didn't hurt as much as I thought*, your brain updates the story. The alarm system we talked about back in Chapter 3 quiets down. You build evidence that you're not broken, just deconditioned, and with each small win, your nervous system relaxes, your muscles switch back on, and your pain starts to lose its grip.

Again, the research backs it up. A 2018 study in *Arthritis Care & Research* found that people who were more fearful of movement and less confident in what their body could do had more pain, more disability, and slower recovery, even when their scans looked exactly the same as everyone else's.[35] Think about that for a second. It's not always what's happening inside your joint that holds you back; it's what's happening inside your head.

Take Lynda, for example. When she first came into the clinic, she couldn't straighten her knee and was convinced surgery was inevitable. We worked through the three movement steps: loosening, nudging, and locking in, but the biggest change wasn't in her leg – it was in her mindset.

The first time she climbed the clinic stairs without holding the rail, she stopped halfway, laughed, and said, 'I can't believe how easy that felt.' That's the moment fear lost, and confidence won.

That's the real goal of this chapter: not just to move freely, but to trust your body again.

The way out of the pain cycle

If pain is what stopped you, movement is what restarts you. By now, you've seen what happens when stiffness eases up, you move better, your confidence grows, and your body starts to trust itself again. That's huge progress.

Here's where most people go wrong. They stop there. They think, *I'm moving better, I'm done.*

You're not done. You've just opened the door, because once you've regained movement, you've got to keep it. The only way to keep it is by protecting it with strength.

Strength is what holds the whole system up. It's what allows function to return, what makes mobility smooth, and what brings the capacity to keep going day after day. Without it, every movement feels harder, every joint takes more strain than it should, and the vicious cycle rolls on.

This is exactly where so many people with arthritis get stuck. They chase pain relief instead of chasing strength. Painkillers, gels, ice packs, and even surgery can quiet the symptoms, but they don't rebuild the system.

The research is clear – people with arthritis who build muscle strength (even gradually and starting from a low base) report less pain, greater confidence, and more freedom in daily life than those who don't. One large review found that strength training cut arthritis pain scores by up to 40%.[36]

One of my patients couldn't walk for more than five minutes without knee pain. After a few weeks of targeted strengthening, they were back to strolling around the shops. Nothing changed on their scan.

Their muscles simply started doing their job again. As they put it, 'I thought I'd just have to survive with arthritis. Now I feel like I'm living again.'

That's the power of rebuilding strength: the difference between surviving with arthritis and actually thriving with it. If you take one lesson from this chapter, let it be this: pain isn't the goal – strength is. The stronger you are, the more your joints are protected, the more freely you can move, and the more of life you get back.

That's why the next chapter is so important. We'll get specific on exactly how strength relates to pain, how to build strength safely with arthritis, what really works, what to avoid, and how to find the right balance between pushing enough and not pushing too far.

Strength isn't just another therapy option for arthritis – it *is* the therapy!

Here's something most people don't realise – as soon as you start freeing up a joint, the muscles around it wake up. Mobility and strength aren't two separate boxes to tick; they feed each other. In fact, the best progress happens when you mix both: a few minutes loosening a stiff joint, followed by some strength-building activity that teaches you how to move again.

For example, if you've been working on knee mobility with a heel-prop stretch, the next step isn't more stretching; it's adding a small muscle engagement called an isometric hold. Relax – we'll talk about this in the next chapter, but simply, it means tightening the thigh muscles as the leg straightens and holding it for a few seconds. It's a subtle but powerful way of teaching the muscle to take back control from the joint.

This is where the next chapter picks up: how to build strength safely, step by step, once your movement starts to return. You're unlocking your body's potential again. Now it's time to protect it – with strength.

5
Rethinking Strength

If movement gets you through the door, strength is what builds the walls around it. Now that your joints are starting to move more freely, the next step is teaching your muscles to take over the job your joints have been doing alone, because without strength, that new mobility won't last.

Most people with arthritis have the wrong picture in their heads when they hear the word 'strength'. They imagine sweaty gyms, bodybuilders with bulging biceps, or Olympic weightlifters dropping bars on the floor. No wonder so many think, *That's not for me/I'm too old/It'll only make things worse,* but what people don't realise is that strength has nothing to do with bodybuilding and everything to do with joint protection.

Strength is the body's insurance policy. It's what keeps your knees from buckling when you step off a kerb. It's what lets you get up from the sofa without using your hands. It's what allows you to lift your grandchild or carry the shopping without bracing for pain.

Think of it as your armour against arthritis. Stronger muscles mean less pressure on sore joints, better balance, and more confidence that your body won't give way, because strength isn't about lifting more; it's about living more.

Take Maggie, one of my patients in her late sixties. She came to me convinced her arthritis meant the end of her active life.

'I thought weights were for young people,' she said when we talked about strength. 'Every time I try to do more, my knee flares up.' What she didn't realise was that the very thing she was avoiding, movement, was the key to getting her life back.

We started small, with basic sit-to-stands, step-ups, and gentle resistance all within her pain tolerance. Within weeks, her legs began to take the strain instead of her knees carrying it alone. Her X-rays hadn't changed, but her life had. She could walk further, climb stairs confidently, and garden again without fear.

A major 2025 review published in the *British Medical Journal* looked at over 15,000 people with knee arthritis across more than 200 studies.[37] It found that structured exercises, especially programmes that focused on strength, led to big improvements in pain and movement in those who followed them, compared to people who just rested or stretched. In other words, the research confirms what I see every day in clinic: when you get stronger, you hurt less and move better, and even if your scans don't change one bit, your life does.

That's the real power of strength. It doesn't just build muscle; it rebuilds trust. Trust that your knees will hold. Trust that your hips won't buckle. Trust that your body won't let you down when it matters most.

Let's be clear from the start. Strength isn't optional; it's the medicine. Without it, function, mobility, and capacity all decline. With it, you don't just move better, you get your independence back.

Before you roll your eyes and remark, 'Easy for you to say, but it hurts when I move,' let's talk about that, because it is the part that keeps most people stuck. Not the pain itself, but what they believe it means.

Should I still exercise if it hurts?

One of the first questions I hear when people start building strength is, 'What if it hurts?' It's a fair question, but it's one that stops most people before they even get started.

When you've lived with arthritis for years, pain becomes the enemy. You've been told to avoid it, to rest when you feel it, to be careful. That sounds sensible until you realise that avoiding pain completely also means avoiding progress.

Let's start with the big one – pain vs damage. Most people have never actually been told this, but feeling a bit of pain doesn't always mean you're causing harm. In fact, when you're rebuilding strength with arthritis, a little discomfort is not just OK, it's normal.

If that sounds hard to believe, a large review by Filipe Raposo et al (2021) published in the *British Journal of Sports Medicine* found that people with knee arthritis who exercised regularly reported significant reductions in pain and improved function even when the activity caused mild discomfort.[38] In other words, discomfort didn't mean harm; it often signalled healing and progress.

It gets better. A study in the *Arthritis Care & Research* journal (2024) showed that a bit of movement-related discomfort can actually switch on your body's own pain-control system.[39] The researchers explained that this kind of discomfort helps activate the body's natural pain-inhibiting pathways, effectively retraining pain sensitivity and reducing overall pain levels over time.

In plain English – remember that over-sensitive alarm system from Chapter 3? Safe, gentle movement helps quiet it down again. That's when your muscles start doing their job properly, and pain begins to fade.

Instead of stopping at the first twinge, you need to understand what the twinge really means, because the challenge now is finding how far to go. Push too little, and nothing changes. Push too hard, and you flare things up.

How do you find that middle ground, the just right zone where progress happens safely? That's where my simple 1–10 rule comes in.

The 1–10 rule

One of the easiest ways to know what's safe when you start exercising with arthritis is to use a simple 1–10 scale, not as a pain score, but as a guide to find your sweet spot for progress.

Here's how I explain it to my patients:

- **1–4 out of 10** is mild discomfort; this is your go zone. You might feel tightness, warmth, or an ache that eases as you move. That's your body saying, 'I'm working, but I'm OK.'

- **5–7 out of 10:** Be cautious here. You can still move, but you'll want to tweak things, maybe reduce the load, slow the pace, or even shorten the session.
- **8–10 out of 10:** That's your red zone. It usually means your body is asking for a different approach.

Your goal is to spend most of your time in the 1–4 range, where you're challenging your body just enough to stimulate strength without setting off a flare-up.

Before, during, and after

Now that you know your range, the next step is learning when and how to pay attention to it. That's where the before, during, after checks come in. This is a simple three-step way to monitor your pain and keep you safely on track:

- **Before:** Is your pain calm enough to start? Below 5 out of 10? If yes, you're good to go.
- **During:** Is it steady or easing as you move? That's a good sign you're in the right zone.
- **After:** Has it settled within twenty-four hours? Perfect. That means your body's adapting.

If pain spikes or lingers for a few days, that's feedback, not failure. Your body's simply saying, 'That was a bit much,' so you adjust; you do not stop.

Sometimes, even with the best plan, your pain will flare or feel unpredictable. That's OK. It doesn't mean you've gone backwards; it means your body's asking for a different kind of movement.

When in doubt, don't stop. Move differently.

Even if your pain feels high (8, 9, or 10), there's always something you can do. That might mean small unloaded muscle activations, gentle chair exercises, or guided electrical stimulation tools (like the new device that we'll talk more about later in the book).

The goal is simple: keep your muscles switched on, because the moment they switch off, your joints are forced to take more of the strain. That's when the cycle of pain starts again.

In fact, a review by the National Institute of Health and Care Research (NIHR) found that people with OA who stopped exercising because they were scared of pain actually did worse than those who kept moving with the right guidance.[40] The ones who stayed active ended up with less pain, less stiffness, and a lot more confidence in their bodies. That's exactly what I see every day in clinic: the people who move, even gently, get better. The ones who wait for pain to disappear first rarely do.

Here's the golden rule: a bit of pain won't kill you, but doing nothing might. Your goal isn't to get rid of pain completely; it's to get strong enough and confident enough that pain stops calling the shots.

The four building blocks of strength

By now, you already know what pain does: it confuses your body, makes muscles switch off, and leaves your joints to take all the strain.

Let's move past the why and focus on the how. This is where you start rebuilding your body, teaching it to move with confidence again and giving those joints the protection that they've been missing.

Strength isn't gained by chance. It's gained in stages. Each stage builds on the last: a little more power, a little more stability, and much more trust in your movement.

Step 1: Activation – waking up the system

You don't need to wait until everything moves perfectly before you start getting stronger. The two grow together.

Once a joint begins to loosen, the next step is to switch its supporting muscles back on. That's what activation does: it connects the mobility you've regained to the strength that will keep it.

Forget fancy machines, forget ten rep maxes. This isn't about lifting heavy weights; it's about reconnecting the system that's fallen asleep.

If pain has been around for a while, your brain has probably turned down some of your key stabilisers: the muscles that should be protecting your hips, knees, and core with every step. Your first job isn't to load them, it's to wake them up.

Activation consists of simple, precise, pain-free movements that switch the right muscles back on and restore timing around your joints. These small isometric holds, roughly ten seconds at a time, aren't about building bulk; they're about control. An isometric hold means tightening your thigh, for example, with a small knee bend, holding an inner range quad contraction, squeezing your glutes, or doing a glute bridge hold. You can see exactly how to do these in the Vault.

These might look simple, but they're doing something powerful: they're waking up stabilisers that pain has silenced. Each repetition reminds your body how to share the load again. That's what sets the foundation for real strength.

A 2021 review in *Frontiers in Physiology* found that the kind of gentle holds and contractions we're talking about, like isometric training, improved joint stability, coordination, and pain in people with arthritis, even before any visible changes in muscle size occurred.[41] In other words, you don't build strength by pushing harder; you build it by reconnecting first. When the system wakes up, strength follows naturally.

This is your starting line: no equipment, no risk; just rebuilding communication between brain and muscle. Once that connection's back, you're ready to move from activation to resistance, because the moment those muscles start firing again, that's when strength, stability, and confidence begin to return.

Step 2: Light resistance – teaching your muscles to take load

Once those muscles are awake, it's time to start using them properly. This is where a light resistance comes in – bands, small weights, or even a tin of beans will do.

You're not trying to lift heavy weights here; you're teaching your muscles to move the joint smoothly through its range and carry their share of the load again. That means gentle, controlled movement with resistance: the kind that challenges your body without aggravating it.

Try seated leg extensions or banded knee straightens (where you push the knee back against a band). For hips, standing abductions, gentle bridges, or hamstring curls to balance the system. Each rep teaches your brain and muscles to work together again, to move with confidence instead of caution.

It's not just theory. A major 2024 review and meta-analysis led by musculoskeletal researcher Lim and colleagues looked at twenty-seven studies of more than 1,700 people with knee and hip arthritis.[42] They found that resistance training, even at light loads, made a real difference. People reported less pain, stronger muscles, and easier movement, with benefits showing up in as little as a few weeks.

The researchers explained that strong quadriceps helped the knee absorb load better and made the joint more stable. In their words, 'Resistance training was effective in improving pain, strength, and function by increasing load absorption and stability in the knee joint.'

In simple terms, when your muscles start taking their share of the load again, your joints finally get a break. This is usually the turning point in clinic. Pain settles. People feel steadier, stronger, and more in control. It's the moment when they stand up and say, 'Hang on, that didn't hurt like it used to.'

Step 3: Bodyweight strength – bringing it back to real life

Now that the system's switched back on and can take some load, it's time to move like yourself again. This is where strength becomes real; it's not about gym gear or big weights, but about control, coordination, and confidence in how you move day to day.

Forget the fancy stuff. Think sit-to-stands (your everyday squat), step-ups, wall push-ups, mini squats, or gentle lunges – the movements you do every single day without even thinking about it. These are the exercises that get your hips, knees, and ankles working together again, the way they're supposed to. Do them right, and they don't just make you stronger; they make movement feel easier. You stop creaking out of the chair, stop wincing on the stairs, and start feeling smoother, more in control.

The research couldn't be clearer. A big *British Medical Journal* review in 2025 looked at thousands of people with arthritis and found that simple bodyweight exercises, things like sit-to-stands and step-ups, did a better job of improving balanced walking speed and everyday confidence than stretching or machine-based workouts.[43] Real-life movement builds real-life strength.

That's why this stage matters, because when you can move your own body smoothly and confidently again, that's when everything changes. The next step is all about turning that strength you've built into freedom, so you can move how you want, when you want, without thinking twice.

Step 4: Everyday strength – turning rehab into real life

Finally, the fun part. This is where all the effort really pays off, because it's not about perfect form in a physio room; it's about proving to your body that it can trust itself again.

Now we move beyond isolated exercises and reconnect everything – muscles, joints, balance, and confidence – so your movement becomes automatic again. Every lift, reach, and step reminds your body, 'I've got this.'

You start applying your strength to real life – carrying the shopping without wincing, climbing stairs without gripping the rail, kneeling in the garden and standing back up with ease, or lifting your grandkids without hesitation. That's what strength is really for – not bigger muscles or personal bests, but freedom. The freedom to move naturally, without bracing for pain or planning every step in advance.

The science backs it up. A 2025 *British Medical Journal* review looked at over 300 trials and found that the biggest improvements in pain relief, confidence, and independence came from functional exercises, the kind that mimic real life.[44] Movements like standing, stepping, and reaching aren't just good for strength; they retrain the brain and nervous system to move smoothly and instinctively again.

In other words, when you practise real-life movement, you build real-life freedom. That's the moment people tell me, 'I stopped thinking about every step, I just moved,' and that's when you know you're no longer rehabbing, you're living.

When you rebuild movement the right way, from freeing a stiff joint, to switching the right muscles back on, to moving confidently in real life, everything clicks. The pain settles, strength builds, and your body starts doing what it was always designed to do.

Let's bring it all together. Here's the roadmap I use every day in clinic, the same process that helps people move from stiff, sore, and stuck to strong, steady, and free again:

1. **Reconnect** – wake up the muscles with inner range holds and activations.
2. **Resist** – use bands or light weights to teach the muscles to take load.
3. **Rebuild** – use bodyweight exercises to restore smooth, coordinated movement.
4. **Integrate** – apply that strength to everyday life.

Each step builds on the one before it. Skip a step, and you'll stay trapped in the same old cycle of flare-up, frustration, and fear. Follow the process, and you'll be amazed at how quickly your movement and your confidence come back. That's how Urban Body helps people not just manage arthritis, but move beyond it.

Here's the question most people have once they get started: 'How hard should it feel?' Push too little, and nothing changes. Push too hard, and you'll flare things up. That's where the next piece of the puzzle comes in: finding your just-right zone, the sweet spot where progress happens safely and consistently. Think of it like adjusting the volume on a radio. Too low, and nothing gets through: the muscles don't get the signal. Crank it up too loud and everything distorts: your joints flare up, confidence drops, and you're back to square one. When you find that middle setting, the signal comes through clearly.

Fine… but how do you know where that zone is?

In practice, it usually means that your muscles should feel challenged, but the joint should feel stable. A bit of muscle effort or mild discomfort during the exercise is acceptable. Pain that lingers, builds as you go or feels worse the next day is a sign you've pushed too far.

Once people understand how to train in that just-right zone, it's not motivation that holds them back, it's misinformation. They've been told what not to do for years until they're scared to do anything at all.

Before we go any further, let's clear up the biggest myths that stop people from ever getting strong again.

Strength training myths (and the truth you actually need to hear)

Myth 1: I'll damage my joints if I lift weights

You've probably encountered this one before – I hear it in clinic almost every week. Sometimes it even comes from a well-meaning doctor or friend trying to 'protect' you.

This couldn't be further from the truth. Lifting doesn't damage joints; it protects them. Muscles act like shock absorbers. The stronger your muscles are, the less pressure your joints take. It's not the load that hurts people; it's the lack of preparation for the load. You don't get arthritis from moving too much. You get stiff and sore from not moving enough.

Strength doesn't grind your joints down; it stops them wearing out faster.

Myth 2: I'll just strap it up and get on with it

If a knee sleeve, elbow strap, or a bit of tape helps you move with confidence, use it. There's no medal for suffering through pain. Supports don't make you weak; they buy you time while your muscles catch up.

Think of them as scaffolding, useful while the structure gets stronger, but not meant to stay forever. Use them to move more, not to move less.

If you find you're relying on a brace all day, every day, that's your cue to start replacing it with muscle. A brace can help you get going, but it's strength that keeps you going.

Wear it to help you move today, but make sure you're doing the work so you won't need it tomorrow.

Myth 3: I'm too old for strength training

Let's be blunt, you're not. Your muscles don't know how old you are; they only know whether you're using them or not.

Research proves this. A 2025 review looked at men and women in their seventies and eighties, and found that even after decades of aches, stiffness, and slowing down, the body still responds to the right training.[45] These people built muscle, improved balance, and even reversed signs of frailty. The authors put it perfectly: 'Skeletal muscle retains its capacity for adaptation well into older age.'

I see it every week in clinic. People who once struggled to carry their shopping, kneel down in the garden, or get out of a chair without wincing are now confidently lifting their grandchildren with ease or playing golf, not because their arthritis vanished, but because their strength and confidence came back.

You don't stop moving because you get old; you get old because you stop moving.

Myth 4: I don't want to bulk up

Don't worry, you won't! Building bulky muscles takes heavy weights, high-calorie diets, and years of intense training. What you do here is completely different. You build lean strength – the kind that helps you lift the shopping, get up from the floor, and move with confidence. You won't get bigger; you'll get steadier. You'll look more capable, not more muscular.

You're not training for the mirror – you're training for your life.

Myth 5: I need a gym to get results

You really don't. Some of the best progress I've seen has come from people who train at home with nothing but a band, a chair, and consistency. A gym can help, but it's not the reason people get better. Commitment is. You don't need fancy kit; you need a plan that meets you where you are. That's why every strength routine in this book is built around things you can do in the living room, in your own time, safely and effectively.

You don't need a membership; you need momentum.

Myth 6: I need to see a doctor first

This is one of the biggest reasons people stay stuck. They wait for an MRI, a referral, or someone in a white coat to tell them it's OK to start moving. For most people with arthritis, you don't need permission to move; you need a plan to move safely.

Doctors are brilliant at diagnosing, but they're not trained to rebuild function. That's what physiotherapists do every day in clinic, helping you move with confidence, reduce pain, and get your life back. The longer you wait for the all-clear, the stiffer and weaker things become, and by the time the letter arrives, you've lost weeks or months you could have spent getting stronger.

Stop waiting for permission and start where you are, because the safest, most proven thing you can do to counter arthritis isn't rest; it's progressive movement.

You don't need a referral to get better; you just need to start.

Where you are now and what comes next

At this point in the book, you've built the foundation that everything else rests on. You've learned how to unlock stiffness (Chapter 4), how to rebuild strength safely (Chapter 5), and how to turn movement into confidence again. You should notice improvements. If things don't feel better in six weeks, go and see your doctor, as something else could be going wrong.

While strength training protects your joints from the outside, what you eat determines how they perform from the inside. Food can be your fuel or your fire. It can calm inflammation or quietly feed it. It can help your muscles rebuild or make your recovery harder than it needs to be.

That's where we're heading next. It's time to make sure you're not undermining your body from within.

6

Food As Fuel (And Fire)

You'd be amazed how often I get asked this: 'Is there a diet that fixes arthritis?'

It's a fair question. When you're tired of pain, it's natural to hope there's a food, supplement, or secret meal plan that can turn things around. Unfortunately, there isn't one food that cures arthritis, but there is a way of eating that can tip the balance in your favour.

Inflammation behaves like a slow-burning fire. Bad food throws petrol on it. Good foods help calm it. That's the power of diet. It creates conditions for your body to move, recover, and rebuild better.

You don't fix arthritis with a food list; you fix it by changing the habits that feed it. A few simple, consistent shifts in what you eat can do more for inflammation and energy than any supplement ever could.

In this chapter, we'll break down:

- Why weight and inflammation matter more than 'good' or 'bad' foods
- How to spot what's fuelling the fire in your diet
- The few supplements that actually help (and the many that don't)
- A simple, realistic way to eat that supports strength, energy, and mobility without the nonsense

Let's start with the biggest pain driver of all: **load**. Every extra pound you carry doesn't just change how your clothes fit; it changes how your joints move.

The weight of the issue

Our bodies were built to move: to hunt, gather, climb, and carry. Food was once hard-earned, and every calorie found was precious, so our bodies learned a very clever trick: store energy when they can because famine might come tomorrow.

Fast forward a few thousand years, and that survival wiring hasn't changed, but the world has. Food is everywhere. Movement is optional. The survival system that once kept us alive now keeps our joints under pressure.

Every extra pound of body weight adds roughly four times that pressure through our knees.[46] If you're carrying an extra stone, your knees are carrying four. It's like walking around with a backpack you can't take off. Every step, every stair, every time you get up from the chair, your knees, hips, and back are doing extra work.

At first, your muscles handle most of the load, but over time, the constant strain tires them out. Once they stop keeping up, the joint is left to take the impact alone, and that's when irritation builds, movement tightens, and arthritis moves in. It's not because your joints have suddenly worn out, but because they've lost balance and control.

Pressure on the joint is only part of the picture. Fat tissue isn't just sitting there; it's active. It releases chemicals that stir up inflammation throughout the body, like a low-level fire that never goes out. That's why people often notice that when they lose a bit of weight, their hands or shoulders feel better, even though those joints don't carry their body weight. They're not just lightening the load; they're cooling the system.

Pain makes you move less. Less movement means more weight creeps in, and the extra weight makes pain worse. That's the arthritis trap, and I see it every week in clinic.

That same cycle works the other way around as well. Move a little more, lose a little weight, pain eases, movement becomes easier, and suddenly you're back in charge.

You don't need to lose a huge amount either. Research by Stephen P Messier et al (2013) found that dropping just 5–10% of your body weight, that's about half a stone to a stone for most people, cut knee pain and stiffness by nearly half.[47] That's not just theory, it's data. It shows how a few steady, consistent changes can take real pressure off your joints and calm inflammation from the inside out.

This isn't about dieting or starving yourself; it's about giving your joints a fighting chance. When you ease the load, your body thanks you. Walking feels easier, mornings aren't such a battle, and you start moving with confidence again.

If you really want to protect your joints, don't stop at losing weight; build strength as well. Lighter joints and stronger muscles are the perfect partnership. Lose the weight, reduce the load, and suddenly life gets easier. Gardening, walking the dog, getting up from the sofa, all without the familiar ache holding you back.

You don't have to be perfect; you just have to tip the balance back in your favour, one meal, one walk, one smart choice at a time. This isn't about losing weight to look better; it's about losing weight to live better, with less strain, less pain, and more freedom. That's what really matters.

However, load is only half the story. What you eat can either cool things down or keep that fire burning.

The hidden fire that feeds arthritis

If you've ever wondered why your joints flare up after certain meals, this is where things finally start to make sense. Food isn't just calories, it's chemistry. Every meal you eat sends a signal through your body, and your joints are listening. When the right food goes in, inflammation settles. When the wrong food creeps in day after day, it's like pouring petrol on a slow-burning fire.

Inflammation isn't always the enemy. It's part of your body's early warning system, the built-in response that helps repair damage and fight off infection. A bit of inflammation after a workout or injury is actually a good thing; it's how healing starts.

The trouble comes when that alarm doesn't switch off. When inflammation stays on in the background day after day, it stops protecting you and starts breaking you down instead. That's what happens in arthritis: the fire never quite goes out, and some foods quietly add fuel to it, meal after meal.

Few things feed that flame faster than what's sitting on most people's plates.

Sugar and refined carbs

It's not just about weight gain. Sugar and white carbs, such as bread, pastries, cereal, and even fruit juice, cause quick spikes in your blood sugar. Your body has to fight hard to bring those spikes back down, and that constant battle stirs up inflammation in the background.

The science shows that diets high in sugar and refined carbs raise the same inflammatory chemicals we find inside painful, swollen joints.[48] It's why your knees might ache more after a weekend of treats or takeaways, and that fire doesn't burn out overnight.

Sugar isn't the only culprit hiding in plain sight. Some of the biggest inflammation triggers are the very oils we cook our 'healthy' meals in.

Seed oils and processed foods

Vegetable oil, sunflower oil, soybean oil… they're cheap, they're in everything, and they quietly build up inflammation over time. They're **silent saboteurs**.

Here's why: they're packed with omega-6 fats, which your body turns into inflammatory chemicals. A little of these fats is fine; you need them, but when your body gets overloaded, and you don't balance them with omega-3 (from fish, chia, or flax), that fire gets stuck on high heat (more on this shortly).

It's not just oils. Processed red meats like sausages and bacon can have a similar effect. It's not the meat itself that's the problem; it's the combination of salt, preservatives, and unhealthy fats created during high-heat cooking. Lean, unprocessed cuts of beef, chicken, turkey, or lamb a few times a week are fine, especially if you pair them with colourful veg and olive oil. The trouble starts when processed versions creep in daily.

The ultimate recipe for joint trouble is a burger and a fizzy drink. You've got refined carbs, seed oils, processed meats, and sugar all in one meal – the perfect storm for inflammation. You might not notice it after one meal, but eat this way for months or years, and your joints will feel it. They get puffy and tight, not from overuse, but from the inside out.

Just when you think you've dodged the biggest food triggers, another one sneaks in from a different direction. It's not hiding in your cupboards this time; it's poured into your glass.

Alcohol

Most people don't realise how quickly alcohol, particularly beer, feeds joint inflammation. Beer is high in purines, which raise uric acid, the same compound found behind gout flare-ups, but even wine and spirits can stir things up by dehydrating tissues and spiking inflammation. You might notice it the morning after a drink: hands feel stiffer, knees feel heavier, and there's a dull ache that wasn't there the day before.

It's not about never drinking again; it's about knowing that every extra glass keeps the body's thermostat turned up a notch. Cut back, stay hydrated, and you'll often feel the difference within days – lighter joints, calmer mornings, and a clearer head to go with it.

You can probably see the pattern by now. Most of these foods and drinks don't just irritate your joints directly, they stir things up from the inside, and nowhere is more important than in your gut.

Your gut – the missing piece

Most people think arthritis lives in the joints, but for many, it actually starts in the gut. Around 70% of your immune system lives there, quietly deciding what to fight and what to tolerate, so when your gut lining gets irritated, from processed foods, antibiotics, stress, or low fibre, it can start letting tiny particles leak into your bloodstream. Your body treats those particles like invaders and attacks them. That constant background battle keeps inflammation simmering, and your joints are often the ones to pay the price.

That's why so many people notice that when they clean up their diet, their joints feel calmer even before any weight comes off. They're not imagining it; they're resetting the system, not just soothing the symptoms.

Once you understand what's been fuelling the fire, the next step is to...

Turn down the heat

Inflammation isn't permanent. You can calm it down, you just have to give your body the right materials to rebuild balance.

Let's start with one of the best 'cooling' foods of all.

Omega-3 fats

If you've been living on painkillers just to get through the day, this part matters. One of the best ways to calm inflammation doesn't come in a capsule; it comes on your plate.

Omega-3 fats are nature's anti-inflammatories. You'll find them in oily fish like salmon, mackerel, and sardines, and in plant sources such as chia seeds, flax seeds, and walnuts.

Most people today get far too many omega-6 fats from processed foods and seed oils, and not nearly enough omega-3s to balance them out. As that ratio drifts, the body stays on alert, swollen, sore, and easily irritated. Bring the balance back with more omega-3s, and you start cooling your system down again. It's a bit like turning down a thermostat that's been stuck on high for years.

Big studies show that people who eat more omega-3-rich foods have lower levels of inflammation markers such as c-reactive proteins and IL-6, the same chemicals found in swollen, painful joints. A major study published in *Surgical Neurology* found that patients taking around 1,200mg of omega-3s daily experienced pain relief on par with anti-inflammatory drugs, but without the stomach or heart risks that come with long-term medication.[49] Even better, almost 60% of them were able to cut down or stop their prescription painkillers altogether.

Omega-3s are found naturally in oily fish, so while the study used supplements, making these foods a regular part of your week can deliver the same anti-inflammatory benefits through real food, not tablets. That's how powerful using food the right way is.

If you want to start simple, aim for two portions of oily fish a week. A tin of sardines on toast or a salmon fillet with roasted vegetables is enough to make a measurable difference over time. For vegetarians and vegans, base some of your meals around walnuts, chia seeds, or flax seeds for the same benefits. Many of my patients tell me that within a month or two of eating this way, their mornings feel easier, and they experience less distance stiffness, more movement, and a quieter ache that doesn't dominate the day.

Colourful fruit and veg

The more colour on your plate, the better your joints tend to feel. Those bright reds, deep purples, and dark greens aren't there for decoration; they're doing a job. Each one brings its own set of antioxidants that help clear out bits of damage inflammation leaves behind. This is your body's way of tidying up before things build into a bigger problem.

It's not about living on kale and beetroot smoothies; it's about variety. Add a handful of berries to breakfast, some spinach or peppers to lunch, and a mix of greens or root veg at dinner. Even small increases like these can lower inflammation markers in as little as six to eight weeks.

Olive oil, turmeric, and ginger

These aren't trends, they're tools. Extra virgin olive oil contains a natural compound called oleocanthal, which behaves in a similar pathway to ibuprofen, calming inflammation without the side effects profile.

Turmeric and ginger go one step further. The real power in turmeric comes from its active compound, curcumin, which is what gives it its golden colour as well as its anti-inflammatory effect. Together, turmeric and ginger block inflammatory pathways that drive arthritis and stiffness, but in a far gentler, more natural way than medication.

A 2021 meta-analysis in *Clinical Nutrition* found that regular turmeric (curcumin) intake reduced arthritis pain and stiffness within six to eight weeks.[50] It's not a quick fix, but when people stay consistent, adding a teaspoon into a curry or even scrambled eggs, they often find their joints feel looser and mornings start easier.

Curcumin needs a little help to be absorbed. Combine it with black pepper (piperine) and a source of healthy fat like olive oil or avocado to make sure your body can actually use it. Think of it as turning an everyday spice into a potent anti-inflammatory.

One caveat worth mentioning: most research uses turmeric supplements, not food. If you're on blood pressure medication or blood thinners, avoid capsules unless advised otherwise. Using turmeric as a spice in cooking is a different conversation and is generally well tolerated.

Ginger is often overlooked, but it does a similar job. Used regularly, it helps calm irritated joints and makes movement feel less reactive. In clinic, people may notice easier mornings and less stiffness when ginger becomes part of their routine. Cooking with fresh ginger or having ginger tea most days tends to work better than the occasional large dose.

The balance

You don't need to be perfect; you just need to change the direction of travel. Every small swap – sugar for fruit, fried for grilled, seed oils for olive oil – nudges your body out of inflammation mode and back towards balance.

It's not about perfection or punishment; it's about patterns. When you shift what you do most of the time, your body starts to listen. Inflammation eases. Energy returns. You feel lighter, steadier, more in control.

If you're wondering what the right diet looks like day to day, here's a simple example:

- **Breakfast:** Greek yoghurt with berries, chia seeds, and a drizzle of honey, or a couple of eggs on wholegrain toast with spinach.
- **Lunch:** A salmon fillet or a tin of sardines on toast with mixed salad, olive oil, and lemon.
- **Dinner:** A lean protein like chicken or lentil stew with colourful vegetables, cooked in olive oil, with a handful of nuts or seeds on the side.
- **Snacks:** A piece of fruit, a protein shake, or a handful of almonds instead of crisps or biscuits.

This isn't a diet, it's a rhythm: one that fuels movement, supports strength, and helps your body repair itself. Each choice is like turning the volume down on inflammation and turning the lights back on in your joints. If you want more simple ideas like this, to keep things easy and consistent, I've put together a few options in the Vault.

By this point, if you've been following the advice throughout the chapters, you are likely to notice the difference. Food, movement, and strength take you 80% of the way, but for some, adding a few well-chosen supplements can give that extra 10–20% edge – as long as you use them wisely. Think of them as tools to reinforce what a good diet starts, not to replace it.

Supplements: hope vs hype

If you've ever stood in front of a shelf of arthritis supplements and wondered, *Do any of these actually work?* the short answer is that most of them promise far more than they deliver. That doesn't mean supplements are useless; a few can genuinely help, but most sit somewhere between underdosed, oversold, and unnecessary if your diet and strength are right.

If you've been relying on anti-inflammatories or painkillers just to get through the day, you're not alone. Many people reach the point where tablets help in the morning, but the side effects and long-term risks start to weigh heavily, so is there a safer alternative?

Before we go any further, it's worth saying clearly, I'm not suggesting that you stop or change your medication without speaking to your GP first. What follows isn't medical advice, but a look at what current research is showing so you can make an informed decision for yourself.

Every week, someone brings a bag of bottles into clinic and asks, 'Should I be taking these?' The real question is, what actually moves the needle for joint health?

The few supplements that are worth your money

Turmeric (curcumin)

As we talked about earlier, turmeric's power comes from curcumin, its active ingredient. It works on the same inflammation pathway as drugs like ibuprofen, just without the gut irritation.

If you want a stronger effect than you'd get from food alone, a curcumin supplement can help. Several good-quality studies and reviews show that taking around 500–1,000mg of curcumin a day, especially with black pepper (piperine) and a bit of fat (like olive oil or avocado), can ease arthritis pain and stiffness over six to eight weeks.[51]

It's not instant, but people who stick with it feel looser in the mornings and less irritated throughout the day once it's had time to build up. It's not numbing the pain like a pill; it's calming what's causing it.

If turmeric's the slow, steady cool-down, Boswellia's the next gear. The two work hand in hand, one cooling the fire, the other keeping it from flaring back up.

Boswellia serrata

You've probably never heard of it, but Boswellia comes from the same tree as frankincense – yes, that one from the Christmas story. It helps to switch off one of the main inflammation triggers in your body, so the joints don't stay stuck in that swollen, irritated state.

It's been used for centuries to calm pain and swelling, and studies are showing why it works so well. A big 2018 review found that people with knee arthritis who took Boswellia had less pain and better movement within a few weeks.[52]

It's even better when paired with turmeric, with which it works hand-in-hand. One is cooling the fire, and the other is stopping it from flaring back up.

If you want to try it, go for a standardised extract (100–250mg a day) and take it with food. It's generally safe, but always check with your GP if you're on other medications.

After taking Boswellia supplements for a few weeks, patients often tell me it's the first time their joints have felt calm in the morning for a long time. The pain is not gone completely, but the joints are easier, with less of the stiffness that used to start their day.

Herbs like turmeric and Boswellia work locally to cool inflammation in the joints themselves, but if you want to take that effect further, calming inflammation throughout the whole body, not just where it hurts, that's where omega-3 fats come in.

Omega-3 supplements

If you don't eat fish or struggle to get enough omega-3 through food, that's where a supplement can bridge the gap. The two key fats you're looking for are eicosapentaenoic acid (EPA) and docosahexaenoic acid (DHA). They're the real workers here; they calm the same pain-triggering chemicals that ibuprofen targets, just without the stomach trouble or heart risks that come with long-term tablets.

Most people do well with about 1,000 mg of combined EPA and DHA per day. If your joints are already hot and swollen, going a little higher, up to 3,000mg, can help even more, but check with your GP before you change anything.[53]

The benefits don't stop at your joints. Omega-3s help blood flow, muscle recovery, and even brain sharpness. Plenty of people tell me that after a few weeks of taking omega-3 supplements, they feel clearer in the head, steadier in the mood, and less foggy throughout the day. That's no coincidence, as DHA fuels your brain just like it does your joints.

If you do buy a supplement, buy well. Go for a triglyceride form of fish oil, with proper third-party testing (like IFOS certification). That way, you know it is fresh and potent. Skip the bargain bottles on the supermarket shelf; they've often sat there too long, and once oil oxidises, it loses its power before you've even opened the lid.

Omega-3s won't work overnight, but they're one of the few supplements I genuinely trust. They're safe, proven, and they help your body do what it's designed to do – heal, not hurt.

Once you've cooled the inflammation, the next step is to support the structure itself: the cartilage, tendons, and ligaments that keep your joints stable and moving smoothly. That's where collagen comes in.

Collagen peptides

Collagen supplements are having their moment right now. Adverts promise they can rebuild cartilage or turn back the clock on your joints. If only it were that simple.

Collagen is the protein that holds you together; it's your cartilage, tendons, ligaments, and skin. Think of it as scaffolding; it keeps everything strong, flexible, and resilient. As you age, that scaffolding starts to weaken, and your body makes less of it.

For a long time, experts thought collagen supplements couldn't help because the molecules were too big to be absorbed properly, but that changed when newer studies looked at hydrolysed collagen – a smaller broken-down form your body can actually use. A 2019 review by Juan Mario García-Coronado and colleagues found that daily hydrolysed collagen reduced pain and improved movement in people with knee arthritis.[54] More recently, a large systematic review by Brueckheimer et al looked at dozens of clinical trials that showed the same effect in both older adults and young athletes – better mobility, less pain, and signs of improved cartilage health.[55]

The key appears to be consistency and dose. Around 10–15 grammes a day, taken with a source of vitamin C (like orange juice, berries, or a supplement), seem to help your body make more of its own collagen. People often say their knees feel more stable or their joints a little stronger after a couple of months of taking collagen, not because it's rebuilding cartilage overnight, but because it's improving the environment their joints need to heal.

Quality matters here. Cheaper powders can be contaminated or underdosed, so stick with brands that publish third-party testing, and remember: collagen alone won't fix an inactive lifestyle. It works best alongside strength training and a good diet, the things that help your body actually use what you give it.

Some people swear by collagen, others think it's a waste of money. The truth is somewhere in the middle, but if you're eating well and staying active, it can give your joints a bit of extra support. It's not going to rebuild what's already worn, but it can help the system run a little more smoothly.

If you'd like to get the benefits of turmeric, collagen, and Boswellia in a simple way, here's a blend I've shared with hundreds of patients. It's become part of their morning routine, and I call it the **Golden Drink**.

Here's what you need:

- 1 tablespoon turmeric powder (curcumin)
- 1/2 mug hot water
- 1/2 mug unsweetened coconut or oat milk
- A pinch of black pepper to boost absorption by up to 2000%
- Optional: 1 scoop collagen powder

Combine the ingredients, stir until the mixture turns a rich golden colour, and sip it slowly in the morning before pain and stiffness have a chance to build.

The warmth helps loosen stiff joints while the turmeric and collagen give your body what it needs to settle inflammation and start repairing. You can find easy-to-follow instructions in the Vault.

If you're also using Boswellia, this is a perfect time to take it. It and the Golden Drink work well together as a two-step system that cools inflammation and supports cartilage at the same time.

It's not a miracle drink, just a simple, practical way to give your body what it needs to settle things down. Stick with it for a few weeks and you'll likely notice the difference: less morning stiffness, easier movement, and a quieter ache that no longer dominates the day.

Once inflammation is under control, your body needs the right building blocks to repair what's been worn down. That's where protein makes the difference: it's the fuel for recovery, not just maintenance.

Protein powder (the overlooked essential)

Protein isn't just for gym-goers. It's the raw material your body uses to repair and rebuild muscle, tendon, and cartilage: the very tissues that protect your joints.

Most people over fifty simply don't eat enough protein. Research shows older adults often consume 25–40% less protein than they need to maintain strength and joint stability.[56] When protein runs low, muscles lose their ability to absorb impact. More load shifts to your joints, and pain creeps back in.

That's where a simple protein supplement can help. It's not about bulking up. It's about giving your joints back-up. A daily shake made with whey or a high-quality plant blend gives your body the amino acids it needs to stay strong. Whey protein in particular is rich in leucine, which switches on the body's repair process.

A major 2023 meta-analysis found that higher protein intake (1.2–1.6g per kg of bodyweight) significantly improved strength, balance, and mobility in adults over fifty, especially when combined with resistance training.[57] That combination, protein plus strength, is what truly keeps joints healthy.

How much do you really need? For most people over fifty, aiming for around 80–100 grammes of protein a day is a good, realistic target. Spread it out across meals: eggs or Greek yoghurt at breakfast, chicken or fish at lunch, beans or lentils at dinner, and a quick shake if you're in a rush.

When patients start hitting those numbers consistently, they often tell me their legs feel steadier, and they recover faster after walks or workouts. They don't notice it overnight, but one day they realise they're moving with more confidence and less effort.

Protein powder isn't about storing anything. It's about giving your muscles what they need, day after day. Regular protein intake supports muscle repair, helps maintain the tissues that protect your joints, and improves how well your body tolerates load. Pair it with movement and strength work, and you'll feel the difference in how your body moves, not just how it looks.

Protein gives your body the materials to rebuild, and creatine gives it the power to use them.

Creatine – the hero for strength and joint protection

Creatine is a natural compound your body makes from amino acids, the same building blocks found in protein. It's stored in your muscles and brain, where it helps produce quick energy for movement and mental focus.

It isn't a joint supplement in the traditional sense, but it's one of the most effective for joint protection. By helping your muscles hold more energy, it allows them to work harder for longer, meaning they absorb more load.

Creatine helps older adults maintain muscle mass and power, which takes the pressure off the joints and improves balance. Research from the *Journal of Gerontology* 2021 found that resistance training plus creatine led to significantly greater gains in strength and mobility than training alone.[58] Stronger muscles mean better support, less fatigue, and more confidence in how you move.

It doesn't stop there. Recent research shows that creatine is not just for muscles. A study in *Scientific Reports* found that a single dose of creatine enhanced brain energy markers and processing speed in sleep-deprived adults, highlighting creatine's role in supporting brain metabolism as well as muscle performance.[59]

For most adults, 3–5 grammes a day is ideal. It's tasteless, safe, and easy to stir into water or a morning shake. Think of it as a small daily habit that keeps you steadier, stronger, and sharper – protection from the inside out.

Supplements can support your recovery, but they can't replace it. Think of them as the extras, useful once the fundamentals are in place – movement, strength, and balanced nutrition will always do more for your joints than any capsule on a shelf.

As I tell my patients, you can't supplement your way out of a bad diet or an inactive lifestyle. Get the basics right first. The supplements come later, and only a few of them are worth keeping.

What about glucosamine and chondroitin?

These two are everywhere. You'll find them stacked high in chemist and supermarket aisles, promising to rebuild cartilage and ease arthritis pain.

Do they work? In short, sometimes, but not for everyone and not as much as the marketing suggests.

Glucosamine is a natural compound found in cartilage, the cushioning tissue inside your joints. The idea is that if you take it as a supplement, you might top up what's missing, which sounds logical, right? Unfortunately, large studies don't tend to back this up. A major review found that glucosamine and chondroitin only gave small improvements in knee pain for some people who often took months to show any difference at all.[60]

That doesn't mean glucosamine is worthless. Some people do feel a benefit, usually those with mild to moderate knee arthritis who take it constantly for at least three months, but the effects are modest. The reason for variation probably comes down to the type of supplement used (there are different chemical forms) and the dose.

If you want to try it, look for glucosamine sulphate (not hydrochloride) at around 1,500mg daily, ideally combined with chondroitin. As always, check with your GP first if you take medication like blood thinners or have diabetes. Glucosamine can affect how your body handles sugar and blood chemistry.

Glucosamine isn't the miracle it's sold as, but it's usually harmless enough. Like all supplements, it's only worth trying once you've nailed the basics. Think of it as a top-up, not a solution.

When you start eating in a way that cools the fire instead of throwing fuel on it, your whole body responds. Your energy lifts. Your joints don't scream at you first thing in the morning.

If you need a direction to aim for, simply look at the Mediterranean diet. Not the Instagram version with endless pasta and wine, but the traditional one built on colourful vegetables, beans, olive oil, nuts, and herbs. If you're not vegan or vegetarian, it also includes oily fish and small portions of lean meat. Yes, and dairy.

It's the most researched, most realistic anti-inflammatory diet we have. Study after study shows that the Mediterranean way of eating calms inflammation, protects the heart, and helps people with arthritis move better and feel less pain.[61] When the inside settles, the outside follows. Swelling goes down. Stiffness fades. Muscles start working the way they're meant to again.

My final note on food is to think 80/20 – no one eats perfectly all the time. You just need to get it right 80% of the time; that's when you start winning.

Now you understand how food fuels change. It also allows your body to maintain itself, and that's what we're looking at next. It's time to explore the thing that almost everyone overlooks: recovery.

7
Constant Recovery

Your body isn't wearing out, it's working overtime.

It surprises people when we talk about this in clinic, but your body isn't giving up on you at all. In fact, it's trying to heal you, constantly, all day and all night, whether you support it or not. Once you understand that, recovery starts to make a lot more sense.

Most of us grow up thinking recovery is something that happens at the end of everything else – after the day settles, after the house finally quietens, after you collapse on the sofa and hope your joints stop nagging – but recovery doesn't wait politely for you to finish your to-do list. It's always running in the background, repairing micro-damage, calming inflammation, settling your nervous system, patching up the muscles you asked a bit too much of, and preparing your joints for another go tomorrow.

Once you reach your fifties, that recovery system still works brilliantly; it just doesn't absorb pressure the way it used to. It's slower to reset, easier to overwhelm, and far less forgiving when you push through tiredness, stress, or broken sleep. None of this means you're fragile. It simply means the system needs more support than it did in your twenties – support that most people don't think about until things start to go wrong.

People never come into clinic saying, 'Phil, my recovery system is exhausted.' They come in saying things like, 'My joints are wearing out,' 'I must have slept funny,' or 'My arthritis is getting worse again,' but when we dig into their week – the broken nights, the long periods of sitting, the low hydration, the background stress they barely acknowledge – a different picture appears. The joint isn't failing. The recovery system behind it is running on fumes.

When your recovery system is tired, everything takes a bit more out of you than it should. Strength doesn't build so well. Mobility you gained yesterday slips away by morning. Even a gentle walk feels heavy, slow, and strangely hard. Little niggles become bigger ones. You wake feeling older than you did the day before.

People see this as deterioration. I see it as under-recovery.

Think of your body as running two shifts:

1. The day shift keeps everything ticking over: hydration, circulation, hormones, movement, posture, and stress.
2. The night shift steps in to repair the mess the day left behind, clearing inflammatory chemicals, restoring pain thresholds, stitching tiny bits of damage back together.

In your twenties, both shifts were fully staffed. In your fifties and sixties, those staff still show up, just under-fuelled, sleep deprived, and trying to juggle too many jobs at once. Your day shift is running dry, your night shift arrives late and leaves early, and your nervous system – the manager of the whole place – is often working in a state of quiet panic.

This chapter is about getting those two shifts back on your side. Not with gadgets. Not with hacks. Not with injections or miracle creams, but with the basics, done consistently, intentionally, and with an understanding of what your body is already trying to do.

Why recovery matters more after fifty

Once you're past fifty, you don't have the same buffer you had in your twenties. Back then, you could get away with late nights, long days, stress, rubbish sleep, and still wake up more or less fine. Now? One or two bad days and your recovery is already behind. You feel it fast: stiffness that won't shift, strength that doesn't stick, and joints that act older than you really are.

I had a man in his early sixties come into clinic recently, convinced his knee had gone downhill overnight. He was genuinely worried. We checked everything – movement, strength, swelling – and nothing had changed. In fact, he'd improved!

Then he mentioned, almost casually, that he'd been living on four to five hours a night of sleep all week because of a work deadline. That was it. Not deterioration. Not joint damage. Just an exhausted recovery system.

When recovery falls behind, your joints feel worse, even when nothing structural has changed. The good news is that once you support the recovery system, your symptoms usually settle faster than you might expect.

Your recovery system has plenty of moving parts, but in my experience, three levers do the bulk of the work. Get these right, and everything else starts behaving: your joints, your energy, your confidence. Miss them, and you spend your days wondering why progress keeps slipping through your fingers.

I call the three levers the Recovery Triangle.

The Recovery Triangle

Three simple levers, 80% of the impact, and the first one is by far the most powerful.

Lever 1: Sleep

Sleep is likely the most underused painkiller you have. Once you're past fifty, it becomes one of the biggest deciding factors in how your joints feel each morning. Not a bonus. Not something you squeeze in if you can. A foundation. The part of your recovery system that holds everything else together.

When someone in their fifties or sixties tells me their pain has suddenly got worse, I don't jump straight to their joints. I ask about their sleep. Nine times out of ten, they look slightly embarrassed before they answer, 'Awful,' or 'Barely any,' or 'Not been great this week,' or 'Up at 3am again,' or my personal favourite, 'I fell asleep on the sofa and woke up wide awake at midnight… you know how it is.'

Yes, I do know how it is, not because it's part of getting older, but because broken sleep is one of the earliest signs that the body's recovery system isn't keeping up anymore. Arthritic joints rarely change overnight. Your recovery does.

What does your night shift actually do?

People think sleep is rest. It isn't. While you're asleep, out of the way, your body clears inflammation chemicals, repairs micro-tears in muscles and tendons, resets your pain threshold, and calms the nervous system back down after the day. It's the night shift clocking in.

There's a study from University of California, Berkeley that gets quoted a lot in my world, and for good reason.[62] It found that after just one night of poor sleep, pain sensitivity increases by around 30% the following day. Your joints don't change, your nerves do. They're simply louder, quicker to react, and more protective. If you string a few bad nights together, the effects compound.

When you've underslept, stiffness feels stiffer, aches feel sharper, flare-ups last longer, and the whole system is running a couple of notches higher on the pain thermostat. The sad part is that people live in this state for so long that they forget what a well-rested body actually feels like.

Why does sleep change after fifty?

It's not your imagination; sleep genuinely becomes more fragile the older you get. You get less deep, restorative sleep. You wake more easily. Temperature affects you more. Noise affects you more. A busy mind affects you more. Yes, the bladder becomes more opinionated than anyone wants.

Layer on late-night screens, partners tossing and turning, hormonal shifts, uncomfortable joints, and general life pressure, and sleep starts taking hits from every angle.

Here's the part I want you to really hear: poor sleep is common, but it isn't permanent. It's responsive. You can aim for improvement, not perfection. You just need conditions your body can actually repair in.

'But Phil… I can't sleep because I'm in pain.' I hear this more than almost anything else, and I get it.

Pain wakes you up → you toss and turn → you get up shattered → you move less the next day → your joints tighten → you go to bed already behind → the cycle repeats. It feels like the arthritis is getting worse. It isn't.

You don't break the loop by lying there hoping for the best. You break it by sending your nervous system the right signals it needs before bed, signals that say, 'We're safe, we can turn everything down now.'

What makes the biggest difference? People often think they need a new mattress, or stronger tablets, or some expensive sleep reset gadget, but the things that help most are almost embarrassingly simple:

- **Light:** Your body is wired to respond to daylight. The day shift switches on with morning light.

The night shift begins when light fades. You don't need to go to bed at sunset or wake at 4am in June. But exposing yourself to natural light in the morning, and dimming artificial light in the evening, helps your body know when to be alert and when to wind down. Late night screens and bright indoor lighting blur that signal, making sleep more fragile.

- **Warmth:** A steaming shower or hot water bottle relaxes tight muscles, guarding a sensitive joint. I've had countless patients who were convinced their night-time pain was bone-on-bone, when really it was tight muscles cramping around an irritated joint. Warmth switches that off.
- **Gentle movement:** Not a workout, but two minutes of slow mobility. Just enough to stop your body going straight from sitting for hours to lying flat with no warm-up.
- **Position:** A pillow between the knees or under the legs can turn five broken hours into a full night's sleep.
- **Switching off:** Often, pain isn't even the culprit; it's adrenaline. If you go straight from TV, emails, or doom scrolling into bed, your body is still wired. You can feel tired and still be nowhere near ready for sleep. Your system doesn't drop from fifth gear to zero on command. It needs a runway, not a crash landing.

If sleeplessness persists, which unfortunately it can do for many people, especially when they get older, there is a valuable resource called cognitive behaviour therapy for insomnia. If you are a resident of the UK, this is available on the NHS and can be a complete game changer, even for people who have tried all the above without success.

'Should I take painkillers before bed?' People ask this as if they're confessing something.

Here's what I tell them. If pain is stopping you sleeping, and your GP agrees it's appropriate, then using pain relief to help you break the cycle is absolutely fine. Sleep is treatment, and if a tablet helps you access that treatment, that's a sensible decision, not weakness. It's a strategy.

Just remember, relying on tablets long-term won't fix anything. They buy time. They don't change the conditions your body is trying to repair.

Poor sleep makes your nervous system more sensitive, your joints stiffer, your inflammation louder, and your recovery slower. It's the invisible force behind countless flare-ups.

When sleep starts to improve, even slightly, the difference shows up quickly. Stiffness eases. Movement feels smoother. Flare-ups lose their intensity. The thing people say most often is simply, 'I didn't feel as bad when I got up this morning.' It's not dramatic, just a small lift that makes the whole day feel easier.

You're not trying to chase perfect sleep or recreate the nights you had in your early twenties. You're simply giving your night shift the fuel it needs to do its job every night, not once in a while.

Once sleep is back on your side, the next lever in the Recovery Triangle becomes far more effective:

Lever 2: Hydration

If sleep is your night-time repair shift, hydration is a member of your support crew that keeps everything running during the day. However, most people treat hydration as something they do to avoid headaches or because it's 'good for' them, and that's usually where the thought process ends. Truthfully, they only remember it on the days someone reminds them they haven't drunk anything since breakfast.

Once you're over fifty, hydration becomes one of the simplest ways to keep your joints calmer, your muscles looser, and your recovery system actually able to do its job. Your cartilage, your discs, your synovial fluid (the fluid that keeps everything gliding), they are all heavily water-based. Not metaphorically. Literally.

When you're running low on hydration, those tissues dry out, stiffen, and lose their spring. That's why you wake up feeling creaky or 'dry' in the morning, or why your legs feel heavier by lunchtime for no obvious reason. Your joints feel dehydrated long before your mouth does.

I rarely meet anyone who's medically dehydrated. That's not what this is. It's the quieter version, the 'I just feel older than I should today' version. In clinic, when a patient and I talk through their hydration day, the pattern is almost always identical: a cup of tea at breakfast, a coffee mid-morning, then nothing until the evening. Not unhealthy or dangerous. Just nowhere near enough fluid for a body that depends on it.

The giveaway moment in clinic is nearly always the same. Someone pauses, thinks for a second, and says something like, 'Well… I did make a tea earlier, but I can't remember if I actually drank it. I left it somewhere.'

Hydration matters more than most people think. Your joints are sponges. When they're well hydrated, they swell slightly, absorb shock, and glide more easily. When they're dry, they become stiff, compressed, and less forgiving. Your muscles feel it too: dry tissues fatigue quicker, tendons tighten, and recovery slows.

People often blame age for that stiff first step in the morning or the feeling that simple movements take more effort than they used to, but for many, it's a body that hasn't had enough fluid to work with. There's research showing that even mild dehydration raises your perception of effort, meaning everything feels hard. One study found that losing just 1–2% of your body's water content can affect mood, energy, and concentration.[63] Anything that affects mood, energy, and fatigue will affect pain.

Over-fifties slide into dehydration without realising it. It happens slowly. Your thirst mechanism becomes less reliable. You avoid drinking to reduce bathroom trips. Water gets replaced with tea, coffee, or diet drinks. Busy days distract you. Some medications increase fluid loss. Most people don't make a conscious decision to drink less; hydration just gets lost somewhere between jobs, errands, and everything else that fills the day.

You don't wake up dehydrated. You just spend long stretches of the day slightly low, and that's when the stiffness, heaviness, and 'one step behind' feeling creep in. You don't need to walk around attached to a water bottle. You need to stop leaving your recovery system to work in a dry environment.

How much should you be drinking?

Hydration isn't a spreadsheet. You don't need perfection. The goal is simply to avoid the long gaps between drinking.

As a rough guide, most people over fifty do well on around a litre and a half to two litres of water across the day. More if you're active, sweating, or it's warm, but consistency matters more than totals. A glass in the morning. Some with meals. A bottle nearby when you're working or out and about. Just enough steady intake that your joints never slip into that dry, heavy stage.

Your body will tell you how you're doing if you pay attention. If your urine is very dark, you're behind. If it's pale yellow, you're generally fine. You don't need apps or trackers – just awareness.

Do tea, coffee, and fizzy drinks count? Short answer: yes, but they can't be the foundation.

Tea and coffee do hydrate you, but caffeine lingers longer once you're over fifty. It tightens muscles slightly, raises heart rate, and nudges your body into a more alert state – not ideal if your system is under pressure. Keeping coffee and tea to early in the day helps.

Fizzy drinks and juices hydrate too, but as previously mentioned, they spike blood sugar and don't support your recovery in the same way water does. Fine as extras, just avoid letting them replace the basics.

Most over-fifties don't notice they're dehydrated until symptoms settle in: that mid-afternoon slump, tighter calves or hamstrings, waking up stiff after a quiet day, feeling unusually hot at night, legs feeling heavier during a simple walk, and a sense that everything takes more effort than it should.

People often say that they just feel a bit older lately without linking it to something as simple as not drinking enough. Understandably, they worry that their arthritis is progressing. In many cases, their body is simply trying to run a recovery system without enough fuel.

What happens when you get hydration right?

Small changes add up faster than people expect. Less stiffness in the morning. Muscles that don't feel as tight. Walking feels lighter. Energy that lasts longer through the day. Sleep often improves too; a well-hydrated body tends to run more calmly at night.

People sometimes describe it as feeling 'lighter' or say that their joints feel 'less sticky', which is a perfect description of tissues working in the fluid environment they're meant to. Your body works better in a fluid environment. Your recovery system works far better in a fluid environment.

Once hydration is sorted, the final lever of the Recovery Triangle becomes much more effective.

Lever 3: Daily movement

If sleep is your night shift and hydration is your support crew, daily movement is the glue that holds the whole recovery system together. It keeps the recovery switched on, but there's one piece people consistently misunderstand – movement isn't about workouts, gyms, or waiting to fix it at the weekend when you've got time. It's small, steady, well-timed bits of movement that stop stiffness from settling in and your recovery system from falling behind.

Most people over fifty think they need more intensity. In reality, their body is begging for more frequency.

When you're younger, you can get away with long sessions of exercise followed by long rest. Your body springs back. Your joints behave. Once you're past fifty, the rules change. Tissues don't love big, heroic efforts; they love rhythm. Predictability. Movement that reminds them what to do rather than shocks them into it.

A study from 2022 found that short, frequent bouts of mobility improved joint lubrication and circulation more effectively than long, infrequent sessions.[64] It's the physiology equivalent of washing the dishes as you go, instead of waiting until Sunday afternoon when you've run out of cutlery.

Your joints prefer little and often to all or nothing, which is why I tell my patients, 'Twenty minutes done most days beats two hours done once in a blue moon.' It's not glamorous, it's not intense, but it works every single time.

People always smile when they hear me use the term 'mobility snacks', as if I'm handing out protein bars, but it's not that. It means doing short bursts of gentle movement, scattered throughout the day. Two minutes here. Three minutes there. Nothing heroic. Just enough to stop your joints from cooling down and your muscles from seizing into positions they'll moan about the next time you stand up.

Things like doing a couple of calf raises while you're waiting for the microwave to ding, balancing on one leg while brushing your teeth (people love this one), and ankle stretches while the kettle boils – these little resets prevent your joints from going on strike. They prevent the slow stiffening that creeps in when you stay still for too long.

The real value isn't the exercise itself, it's the rhythm. Your body responds far better to movement that feels easy, natural, and repeatable; the sort you can slip into your day without thinking.

Of course, take up exercise classes if you want to be more formal about your movement. Yoga and Pilates are both great for arthritis. Yoga eases stiffness, calming the nervous system, and giving your joints a chance to breathe again. Pilates builds the controlled strength around your core, hips, and spine – the strength that stops flare-ups from happening in the first place.

When it comes to movement, most people with arthritis turn their minds to heat packs and ice packs. Both are tools you can use to aid recovery, but there's confusion around how. They're often treated like rival football teams.

'Phil, which one is right?' people ask me. 'Which one actually works?'

The slightly annoying answer is, it depends. Neither one is going to 'fix' the joint, but both can change the environment around it enough for your body to move more and do the repair work itself.

Heat is your go-to when everything feels tight, stiff, or slow to get going. It boosts circulation, relaxes tense muscles, and sends a clear signal to your nervous system that it's safe to turn the dial down a notch. If you wake up creaky, feel like you're moving through treacle, or your back or hips just won't relax, heat is almost always the right choice.

Ice is for the opposite scenario, when something is hot, puffy, or irritated. The classic 'I overdid it yesterday, and now my joint is letting me know.' It calms swelling, dulls pain, and takes the edge off inflammation. Think of it as a temporary mute button, not a cure.

Neither heat nor ice fixes the issue; they change the state your body is in. Heat opens things up so recovery can happen. Ice cools things down, so irritability settles. They're tools, not treatments. Helpful nudges, not solutions, and once you know what each one actually does, the whole decision becomes a lot easier.

Still not sure? Start with heat. It's right more often than it's wrong.

Your recovery routine doesn't need to look impressive. It needs to be predictable. Think of it like brushing your teeth. You don't wait for Friday and scrub them for forty-five minutes. You do a little, often, because that's what keeps things healthy.

Daily movement works the same way. Maybe it starts with a small mobility snack in the morning to wake things up. Later in the day, a short walk, ten or fifteen minutes to reset the system and get the circulation moving again. In the evening, a few slow stretches to stop the day from settling into your joints. Once a week, a class for a bit of structure. When you need it, some warmth on the stiff areas to help things settle.

Nothing perfect, just enough rhythm that your body knows what's coming next. Your joints respond far better to a predictable pattern than to occasional grand gestures, so keep showing up, even on the days you don't feel great, and your body slowly stops guarding and starts cooperating. That's recovery. Not intensity; consistency.

Even when you get this rhythm right, you'll still have days where things feel slightly off. That's where the next part comes in.

When you're doing everything right and still feel off

By this point in the chapter, you may be thinking, *I'm sleeping better, I'm drinking more, so why do I still have days where everything feels off, slow, or one step behind?*

This is the part most people over fifty never look at. Even when the Recovery Triangle is in place – better sleep, better hydration, and more movement – the whole system can still feel off if one of the deeper background settings is dragging its feet. If one part of that network slips, the whole thing slows down long before your joints do.

I'm not asking you to track every metric under the sun; I'm asking you to make sure you're not trying to recover with the handbrake half on. You can be doing all the right things and still feel flat if the foundations underneath aren't supporting the load.

There are three background settings that matter more after fifty than most people realise: your hormones, your circulation, and your resting heart rate.

1. Hormones – the invisible settings

Hormones might not be the first thing you think about when your joints ache, but they influence almost every part of your recovery system. Men see testosterone drift down slowly. Women see oestrogen drop sharply through menopause. Those changes affect far more than mood or hot flushes. They influence how well your muscles repair, how deeply you sleep, how inflamed your tissues feel, how much energy you wake up with, and how sensitive your pain system becomes.

Think of hormones as your body's settings menu, the quiet dials in the background that decide how easily you recover, how well you build strength, and how resilient your tissues feel in day-to-day life. When those settings drift, even slightly, the whole system becomes out of balance.

In clinic, the pattern is almost predictable. Strength is fine… but recovery is slower. Movement is fine… but stiffness lingers. Nothing looks inflamed… but everything feels tired. Sleep becomes lighter. Pain feels sharper, even though nothing mechanical has changed.

It's easy to assume your arthritis is progressing. Often, it's simply that the settings behind the scenes have shifted. This is especially true of women.

You don't need to diagnose yourself or go hunting for treatment, but you do need to know that hormones are part of the recovery landscape. It's worth checking with a medical professional if you feel out of sync for reasons you can't explain.

2. Circulation – the delivery system behind repair

If hormones are your body's settings, circulation is the delivery system. Everything your joints rely on to repair – oxygen, nutrients, warmth, and inflammation clean-up – arrives via blood flow.

Once you're past fifty, that flow naturally becomes less efficient. Not enough to worry your GP, but enough that your body feels the effects before you consciously notice it.

You've probably felt some version of it: the stiff first step in the morning; the cold feet in the evening; legs feeling heavier after days that never used to bother you; a knee that stays puffy long after the activity that caused it. People often blame arthritis, but very often it's simply this: your joints are running on a trickle of blood, oxygen, cells, and nutrients when they used to run on a steady flow.

The fix is not compression tights, vibrating pads, red light socks, or whatever TikTok is selling this week. Circulation responds to things you already know: move more often than you sit, hydrate properly, use your muscles regularly and gently, and strength train, because nothing boosts circulation better.

Think of it like oiling a hinge. Not a deep clean. Not a restoration job. Just the regular movement that keeps everything gliding. When circulation improves, recovery improves, and when recovery improves, joints calm often without you changing anything else.

3. Heart rate – the quiet indicator your body gives you

Resting heart rate is one of the most honest signals your body has. I'm not talking about the number you hit on a walk or during exercise. I mean the number your body sits at when you're doing absolutely nothing.

When your recovery system is in a good place, that number tends to be lower. When you're sleep deprived, under-fuelled, stressed, fighting a virus, or asking too much of your system, it creeps up.

Most people feel the effects long before they ever look at the number. They'll say things like: 'I feel tired for no reason,' or 'I was wired at bedtime,' or 'I woke up feeling like I hadn't slept.'

If someone sits in front of me in clinic and says, 'I don't know what's wrong, I just feel off,' this is one of the first clues I think about. A rising resting heart rate is your body's polite way of saying: 'I'm under load here.'

The good thing is that it responds quickly when you sort the basics out: when you start sleeping a little better, drinking consistently, easing back on caffeine, walking more often, and keeping a calmer evening routine. As resting heart rate drifts down, recovery drifts up, and as recovery improves, pain sensitivity drops, often before anything changes at the joint itself.

That's why I like resting heart rate: it doesn't just tell you about your heart. It tells you how pushed and overwhelmed your whole system is, and one thing pushes that system harder than almost anything else: stress.

Stress – the hidden accelerator of pain

If you've ever had a stressful week and thought, *Why are my joints worse even though I haven't done anything different?* you're not imagining it. Stress is one of the biggest pain amplifiers there is, especially once you're past fifty, but hardly anyone joins the dots. People usually blame age, arthritis, the weather, or sleep not being what it used to be, but when you zoom out, a far simpler pattern appears: the joint often isn't the problem, the system around it is.

Nothing disrupts that system faster than stress. A stressful week → poor sleep → tighter muscles → more inflammation → more pain → even worse sleep. It's a biological loop, not a personality flaw.

Your body reacts to modern stress the same way it would have reacted to real danger thousands of years ago. The threat used to be a sabre-toothed tiger. Now it's inboxes, deadlines, family worries, or a bad night's sleep. A tense phone call or an argument with your partner switches on the same fight-or-flight response your ancestors needed to sprint for their lives. The trouble is, you're not sprinting anywhere. You're sitting in traffic on the M42 or lying in bed staring at the ceiling, while your nervous system behaves as if something big is trying to eat you.

Once you're over fifty, this pattern becomes clearer. A stressful week rolls in, and your joints flare for no obvious reason. A difficult day, and your neck, back, or hips tighten and refuse to switch off. One broken night turns into morning stiffness that feels deeper than usual. Even a busy evening can leave your body wired long after your mind insists you're fine.

None of this is 'in your head'. It's physiology. The wiring hasn't changed, but the triggers have.

One study found that psychological stress reduces deep sleep by up to 20%, and when deep sleep drops, pain sensitivity rises significantly.[65] That's why a stressful week and a flare-up look identical. Stress doesn't break joints; it raises the sensitivity of your entire pain system.

We'll talk about stress in detail in a later chapter on mindset, but when it comes to recovery, it needs to be controlled.

Recovery is a state you live in, not a task you do

The real goal is establishing recovery as a state, not as a one-off task. Most people treat recovery like something they do after they've moved, exercised, gone about their day, gardened, danced, played with their grandchildren, and lived their life. They act like it's a bonus if they've got time, but the body flips that on its head.

Recovery isn't an activity; it's a state your body stays in when you support it. Sleep keeps you in it overnight. Hydration keeps you in it during the day. Movement maintains it. Nutrition strengthens it. Stress pulls you out of it, and pacing your effort pulls you back in.

When recovery becomes a background habit – a way of living, not a programme – everything you do starts working better. Pain drops. Mobility holds for longer. Strength work sticks. Flare-ups calm sooner. Mornings are easier. You feel more like yourself again.

This is the whole point of the chapter. Your body isn't wearing out; it's working overtime. The moment you support it, it responds every single time.

Now we need to talk about the thing people often reach for first, long before they support recovery properly: drugs. In the next chapter, you'll learn how to use medication wisely, without letting it take over the job your body is already trying to do.

8
Drugs

Do painkillers and injections help you or trap you? If they really worked, you wouldn't still be in pain, right?

Most people never question tablets. They're handed them, they take them, and they hope for the best, but here's what I tell patients in clinic every single week: painkillers numb pain – they don't fix what's causing it.

Earlier in the book, I talked about how easy it is to walk out of a GP appointment with a prescription instead of an actual plan. This chapter goes deeper, because tablets don't just change your symptoms, they change your behaviour. That's where you get stuck.

Before we go any further, an important point.

This chapter is not telling you which medication to take, stop, or change. That's your GP's role. My job is to help you understand the patterns I see in people over fifty every single day: how tablets affect recovery, movement, confidence, sleep, and long-term progress.

Please don't alter any medication without speaking to your GP or pharmacist first.

What I want to give you is understanding. Once you understand what tablets are doing to your body and your behaviour, you can make better decisions with your GP instead of just hoping for the best.

The hidden cost of painkillers

On the surface, painkillers feel logical. You hurt, you take a tablet, and the pain drops. Clean, simple and obvious. Except it isn't.

Up to this point in the book, we've been working on the assumption that with less pain, you can naturally do more and have more get up and go. Through the years in clinic, I've learned that this often isn't true.

Pain is exhausting. Once you get a bit of relief, your initial instinct is to rest. Not only that, but medication also has side effects, which can make you feel groggy and in a fog, adding to the level of inactivity.

In my experience, the moment the pain eases, you move less, and when you move less, your strength drops. Once your strength drops, your joints become more sensitive, and when sensitivity rises, the same tablets feel weaker. When tablets feel weaker, you reach for them more often.

By this point, you're not really taking the tablet for the pain anymore. You're taking it for the fear of pain.

That shift usually goes completely unnoticed. It doesn't happen in one dramatic decision. It creeps in. A tablet in the morning 'just in case'. One before a long walk. One after a busy day. One before bed, 'so it doesn't kick off in the night'. One because tomorrow looks full on and you're already worried. Before you know it, the tablet isn't a tool anymore; it's a safety net. Not just for pain, but for everything: movement, sleep, confidence, anxiety, stairs, flare-ups, holidays, gardening, bad days, good days... everything. It's a slow slide from 'This helps' to 'I don't feel safe without it.'

That's how dependence starts. Not addiction, dependence. Just to be clear on the difference, addiction is when you crave a drug, seek it out, and lose control around it. There is well-defined professional help available for addiction. Dependence is much more subtle. It's when your confidence or mood relies on a tablet to get you through the day, even though you never wanted this. There's no craving, just an unintentional drift into feeling like you can't cope without it. Dependency, frustratingly, is less well served.

Most people in long-term pain only realise they are in dependency years down the line, when they finally admit they don't like how many tablets they're taking, but feel terrified to stop. If that resonates, let me say something you've probably never heard from a clinician: 'You weren't born with a painkiller deficiency,' but you'd never know it, judging by the way tablets are handed out on repeat prescriptions with no explanation, no monitoring, and no real plan behind them.

The tablet isn't automatically the villain. The habit around the tablet is where the real damage starts, and that habit feeds the biggest trap people over fifty fall into...

The Painkiller Loop

Here's the pattern I see again and again. I call it the Painkiller Loop.

Pain → tablet → relief → rest → less movement → weaker muscles → louder joints → more tablets.

It always starts innocently. Pain rises → you take a tablet → the pain drops. For a short while, it feels like you've got control back, but once the loop kicks in, everything slows down. You relax, you ease off, and you slip straight back into 'protect the joint' mode.

You might think feeling better would make you move more, but in reality, it often makes you do less. Why? Because the relief feels fragile and you don't want to upset it, so you sit a bit more. You avoid stairs. You skip the walk. Add in the drowsiness or brain fog I have mentioned that stronger medication can cause, and it becomes even easier to move less.

When you move less, your muscles switch off. When your muscles switch off, your joints take more load. More load makes the joint more sensitive. More sensitivity means the pain feels worse the next time it flares, so what do you do?

You reach for the tablet again. A little earlier. A little more often. Just in case. That's the loop.

At some point, you stop trusting your body. You trust the tablet instead. That's the real trap: not the drug itself, but the belief that you can't cope without it.

Used well, tablets create a small window that helps you move. Used badly, they shut the windows, lock the doors, and trap you inside.

This chapter is about breaking the loop, safely, sensibly, and always with your GP involved, so that you can rebuild confidence, not dependence. Let me show you what this looks like in real life.

A woman in her late fifties came to see me with a knee that wouldn't settle. Nothing dramatic. Nothing new. Just a joint that felt unreliable.

She told me, 'I take one tablet first thing in the morning, just to take the edge off.' When I asked her how long she'd been doing that, she gave me that look many people give when they're suddenly realising something themselves. 'I don't know… months? Maybe longer. It started after a bad flare, and now the tablets are part of my daily routine.'

That's the giveaway. Not the pain. Not the arthritis. The routine. She wasn't taking them because her knee was screaming at her. She was taking them because the thought of not taking them made her anxious. Her exact words were: 'I don't trust my knee on its own anymore.'

The loop is not loud or dramatic. It's a slow leak of confidence until the tablet becomes the thing propping you up – not your movement, not your strength, not your own body. When you get to that stage, the tablets stop being the helper and start being an anchor.

The good news is that the anchors can be lifted, and you can break the loop before you break your joints.

When should you use painkillers?

Despite everything I've said, I still use painkillers as part of a plan, and so do good GPs and consultants. Used properly, painkillers have a place. They can break a sharp flare, help you settle enough to sleep, or give you a short relief window where movement feels more manageable.

A painkiller's job is simple: brief relief so you can move. That's it. If it leaves you doing less, waiting for it to kick in, or planning your day around it, it's no longer helping.

Painkillers work best when they create space for you to do the things that actually change your joints: movement, strength, and recovery habits. They stop working the minute you lean on them instead of leaning into your body. That matters even more after fifty, because your body is changing, and so is the way it handles medication.

Why do tablets seem less effective after fifty?

People often say to me, 'These tablets used to ease the pain. Now they barely help. My arthritis must be getting worse.'

Sometimes the arthritis has progressed, but more often, nothing major has changed in the joint. What's actually changed is the system around it: your metabolism, your nervous system, your sleep, your circulation, your other medications, your habits.

Here's what actually changes after fifty:

1. **Your metabolism slows down.** Your system simply breaks medication down more slowly. The tablet needs longer to take effect, and when it wears off, the dip feels more noticeable.

   It's something we see all the time in older adults, but it's rarely explained properly. In plain English, the useful part fades quicker, and the side effects linger longer, so the tablet feels less like a clean on/off switch and more like a dull, unreliable dimmer.

2. **Your nervous system becomes more sensitive.** Studies show that age changes the way your nervous system processes pain signals.[66] It's not more damage, but more sensitivity. It's like your alarm system sits closer to the surface, so normal signals feel louder. That alone makes tablets feel weaker, even if the joint itself hasn't changed much.

3. **Your sleep takes a hit.** You already know from the previous chapter that poor sleep turns the volume up on pain. If you're not getting enough deep sleep, everything feels sharper the next day.

Even if the pain hasn't changed, your experience of it has, and tablets struggle to compete with that.

4. **Circulation slows.** Blood flow changes with age. This affects how quickly tablets get absorbed and distributed. Some days, a tablet works like it used to. Other days, it barely scratches the surface. That inconsistency is normal, but it's rarely explained.
5. **Your brain forms habits quickly.** If you always take a tablet before you move, your brain starts to believe the tablet is what makes movement possible. Not your body. Not your strength. Just the tablet. Once that belief sets in, everything feels harder without the tablet, even if nothing in the joint has changed.
6. **You're often on lots of different tablets, and nobody joins the dots.** By fifty, many people are on a mixture of blood pressure tablets, statins, reflux medication, diabetes medication, the odd sleeping tablet, plus painkillers on top. None of these are bad in isolation, but they're rarely prescribed with each other in mind.

Your heart specialist focuses on your heart. Your diabetes specialist focuses on blood sugar. Your GP deals with whatever problem you walk in with that day.

Everyone means well. Everyone does their job. Almost nobody is looking at the whole picture, so you end up with a mixture of tablets, each with its own timing, side effects, and impact on sleep, sensitivity, and inflammation. Most of the time, nobody is really reviewing this mixture; they're just renewing it.

It's no surprise painkillers feel unpredictable after fifty if your body is already juggling a stack of medications that were never designed to work as a team.

You might recognise this story. A man in his early sixties once told me, 'I feel like the tablets I've been taking for years just stopped working.' When we dug into it, his scan hadn't changed. His X-ray hadn't changed. His diagnosis hadn't changed. What had changed were all the things nobody had joined together: his sleep had been poor for a month, he'd avoided walking because he didn't trust his knee, his quads had weakened, he'd started taking tablets earlier in the day 'just in case', and he was worrying about pain before it even appeared.

His arthritis hadn't suddenly progressed. His whole system had shifted, and nobody had explained how that affected the tablets.

If tablets feel like they've stopped working, it doesn't automatically mean your joints are wrecked. It often means your body has changed, and your strategy hasn't caught up. That's what the next section of this chapter is about: why it is so hard to get off tablets once you're on them, what role the GP systems play in that, and where medication actually fits in.

First, I want you to sit with one key idea from this section:

Tablets are not your only defence. They're one tool in a much bigger plan.

Why do people get stuck on tablets for years?

People don't stay on tablets because they're weak or irresponsible. They stay on them because the system almost guarantees it.

GPs care deeply, but they're working inside a system that gives them ten minutes to fix problems that often took you ten years to develop. This isn't a GP problem; it's a system problem. You walk in with pain, they've got a queue of patients behind you, and they need you functioning enough to leave.

A tablet is the quickest option. 'Try these and come back in six weeks if it doesn't settle.'

On the surface, that seems reasonable, but it creates a different problem. You rarely see the same GP twice. Nobody reviews your medication properly. Nobody checks how long you've been on it. Nobody explains the side effects. Nobody gives you a tapering plan.

Nobody has the time to walk you through how it all fits together.

You end up on repeat prescriptions that drift for months... then years... then decades. Not because you've done anything wrong. Not because the GP doesn't care. It's because the system is overwhelmed, and you get carried along with it.

I see this all the time in the clinic. People are stuck on medications without any idea how they got there or how to get back off of them safely. Let me show you how this plays out in real life.

A woman in her early sixties came to see me. She'd been on tramadol for nearly twenty years, not because she wanted to be, or because her back was getting worse, but because she was frightened to come off it.

Every time she tried to reduce the dose, she felt rough for days: shaky, on edge, unsettled, and the pain seemed to kick off. She didn't know what was true pain and what was her body reacting. She just knew it scared her.

She'd been bounced between her GP and a back consultant for years. The GP told her to ask the consultant what to do. The consultant told her to ask the GP. Each time, the GP she saw was different, so every appointment felt like starting again.

There was no plan, no follow-up, and no joined-up thinking.

She wasn't choosing to stay on the tablets. She just didn't know how to get off them safely, and nobody had ever taken the time to show her. She wasn't addicted. She wasn't weak. She was stuck in limbo, doing the only things she knew: taking the tablets and hoping today wasn't the day everything fell apart.

This is the reality for thousands of people over fifty. Tablets that started as a short-term plan slowly turn into a long-term plan, with no one checking whether they're helping, harming, or simply doing nothing. No one is supposed to manage that on their own, but they end up having to.

Here are the five signs I see in clinic that someone has crossed a line and entered into an unhealthy relationship with pills:

1. They start taking painkillers automatically, the same time every morning, even on days they're not actually in pain.
2. On the days when they've got things planned – shopping, housework, or meeting a friend – the tablet sometimes goes in before they've even tested how the joints feel.
3. When the packet starts to run low, they notice themselves checking their bag or the kitchen

drawer more than usual. That worry isn't really about pain at all; it's about feeling exposed without the tablets close by.

4. They plan their day around the tablet. They time activities for when it kicks in, as if the tablet is the thing that holds them together.
5. They're more frightened of the pain coming back than the pain itself. This is the big one. Once fear drives decision making, movement shrinks, strength drops, and the loop tightens with it.

If this resonates with you, none of this means you're addicted. None of this means you've done anything wrong. It means you've been coping the only way you were shown, but once you see these patterns clearly, you can change them. When you change them, everything else begins to shift: your movement, your confidence, your sleep, your strength.

This is usually the moment where people look at me and ask, 'If I have an injection, does that mean I can finally stop the tablets?' The answer, as I'm sure you suspect, is rarely yes.

Let's look at injections in more detail.

The truth about injections

Most people over fifty I meet don't really know what an injection does. They've heard the usual stories: a neighbour who 'felt brilliant for months' on an injection, a friend who says it changed everything, a footballer who limps through training all week and then magically glides onto the pitch after a quick jab. It all sounds impressive, almost magical, but when you strip away the noise and look at what injections actually do inside your body, the truth is a lot simpler, and far more useful.

First, let's clear up the biggest misunderstanding of all. Footballers are not your point of comparison. People often say, 'If they can have an injection every few weeks, why can't I?' It's because footballers aren't being healed, they're being patched. They've got physios waiting on a touchline, rehab sessions twice a day, massage, ice baths, compression sleeves, doctors monitoring every reaction, and a manager whose job depends on getting them through another ninety minutes… not keeping their joints healthy for decades to come.

They're playing a completely different game. You don't need your knee ready for Saturday; you need it ready for the next twenty years.

When you take footballers out of the equation, you're left with two main types of injection that do completely different jobs. The confusion comes from lumping them together.

Let's examine each one in turn.

Steroid injections (cortisone)

The most common, and the most misunderstood.

People often assume steroids fix arthritis. They don't. They can't reverse damage and they can't rebuild cartilage. What they can do, when the timing is right, is calm inflammation when a joint is stuck in a cycle of irritation and just won't settle. If a joint is hot, swollen, and reactive, the sort where every step feels like pressing on a bruise, a steroid can take that raw edge down. Not permanently, but enough to give you breathing room and space to move again.

The injection itself is a strong anti-inflammatory mixed with a small amount of local anaesthetic. The anaesthetic gives an odd numb feeling for a few hours. The steroid works more slowly over days, calming the irritated joint lining so it stops shouting at you every time you bend or put weight through it.

When the timing is right, that short drop in irritation can feel like someone has turned the volume down from a scream to a level you can actually work with. That opportunity to do the long-term work we've covered earlier in the book is where the research shows the biggest benefit. Most studies agree that the improvement lasts anywhere from two to six weeks, sometimes up to twelve weeks in the right person, and after that it naturally fades.[67]

Here is the part nobody explains. Steroids only help when inflammation is the main driver of pain. If your joint is stiff, dry, crunchy, or simply worn, you might feel absolutely nothing. Not because the injection went wrong or the clinician missed the spot, but because there wasn't enough inflammation for the steroid to act on in the first place.

That's why some people swear by steroid injections, and others shrug and say, 'It didn't touch my pain.' It is also exactly why no steroid injection is ever guaranteed; it only works when the biology actually matches the drug.

Accuracy matters too. Knees are fairly straightforward. Hips and deeper gluteal structures are not. They sit behind layers of muscle, nerves, and blood vessels. The medication has to land exactly in the right place, which is why ultrasound guidance exists. The right hands massively improve the odds of the injection working. The wrong hands can put the perfect drug in the wrong spot and get the same result as doing nothing.

Then there's the long-term worry. Everyone eventually asks, 'Do steroids damage the joint?'

A single injection, used at the right time, doesn't harm the joint; that's backed up by what I see in clinic. The issue comes when the same joint is injected again and again, every few months, year after year, with no strength work or load management alongside it. Some studies show a small but measurable trend towards faster cartilage thinning in those cases – not in everyone and not dramatically, but enough for sensible clinicians to treat steroids as a short-term tool, not a long-term strategy.[68,69]

Even if they're used long term, the real problem usually isn't the steroid itself; it's the lack of anything around it. The joint never gets stronger. The movement never changes. The irritation is treated over and over again, without anyone addressing the cause.

This is the part that matters most: steroids are a reset, not a solution. Used well, they open a small window of opportunity, making movement tolerable again. Used badly, they create the illusion of progress without any real change.

Just so you know where I stand with this: I do use steroid injections, but only in very specific situations. I won't inject just to chase pain away, and I won't inject a joint that's already at the end of its lifespan. If a patient hasn't worked on movement, we fix that first.

Additionally, I won't inject unless there's a clear rehab plan waiting on the other side. If someone keeps needing injections into the same joint, that's usually a sign that something important hasn't been addressed, not a sign they need more steroids.

If your joint is swollen, irritated, and reactive, and you can't move enough to begin strengthening, that's when an injection earns its place. Not as the fix, but as the reset that lets the real work begin.

Steroids aren't the only injection people hear about. The other one, the so-called 'gel injection', gets talked about everywhere from GP surgeries to golf clubs, and just like steroids, it's widely misunderstood.

Let's break that one down properly.

Hyaluronic acid ('gel') injections

If steroid injections are the volume button that turns irritation down, hyaluronic acid (HA) injections are trying to do something completely different. They don't calm inflammation, they don't numb pain, and they're certainly not a stronger steroid.

HA is the same gel-like fluid your joints naturally produce to keep them cushioned and moving smoothly. HA injections are most commonly used in knees, because that's where we have the strongest evidence, but the principle applies to any synovial joint. But after fifty, especially with OA, that natural gel becomes thinner, stickier, and less effective. The joint feels dry, tight, and friction-heavy.

An HA injection aims to top that lubrication back up. It's the closest thing we have for the human body to adding oil to a rusty hinge. You're not repairing the hinge itself, you're helping it move with less resistance.

This is where people often get it wrong. HA helps a very specific type of joint problem. If you say things like, 'My knee feels dry,' or 'It grinds or crunches when I bend it,' or 'It's not swollen, it's just stiff and annoying,' then you're the kind of person HA is designed for. It's for dryness, stiffness, and friction. Not healing, swelling, or irritation.

In short, if your joint is hot, angry, and reactive, steroids help more. If your joint is dry, stiff, and crunchy, HA can make things smoother.

If your joint is inflamed, HA won't help. If your arthritis is very advanced, it won't help, but in mild to moderate arthritis, for the right patient, HA can make movement feel smoother and less clunky for a couple of months. In contrast, others feel absolutely nothing at all.

The research is mixed because people often get HA injections for the wrong reasons. The big *British Medical Journal* meta-analysis found the average benefit is small, sometimes too small to notice.[70] Other studies show meaningful improvement for the right patient, especially with mild to moderate knee OA.[71]

Injections open different types of windows: steroids open a window by calming irritation. HA opens a window by reducing friction. In both cases, the strength you build, the load you improve, the movement you restore is what creates long-term change. The injection isn't the fix. It simply creates the opportunity for the fix.

Injections make change possible, not automatic; the door you choose only matters if you actually move through it. Neither injection changes the joint on its own. Neither rewrites your movement patterns. Neither makes you stronger, steadier, or more resilient.

What should you actually do with all of this?

Painkillers, steroids, gel injections – they can all help, but none of them moves a stiff joint. None of them rebuilds strength. None of them teaches your nervous system to settle or helps your body cope with load again. Those are your jobs, and the good news is that once you take those jobs back, everything else starts to shift.

Medication works best when it creates the conditions for change, not when it replaces the change. Think of it like this: a tablet might help you sleep, but it's the sleep that repairs you. A steroid might calm a flare, but it's movement that steadies the joint. A gel injection might ease stiffness, but strength is what protects you long term. Medication can open a door. What you do on the other side of that door determines what happens next.

What's the plan?

Here's how I guide patients in clinic. It's a simple five-step framework you can follow yourself. It can be in any order that fits with your current situation:

1. **Reset the noise.** Use medication to create a window of opportunity, not as the main strategy. If tablets or an injection help you move better for a few days or weeks, brilliant. Use that window deliberately. That's not the time to rest. That's your chance to build.
2. **Rebuild in the window.** Fill that window with the work that actually changes the joint. Build strength. Keep the joint moving. Improve your sleep. Pace yourself better. Work on the weak spots. This is where almost all of your long-term changes come from.
3. **Relief isn't repair.** No injection fixes arthritis. Anything that wears off was never fixing the joint; it was only calming it.
4. **Get assessed.** If you need repeated medication just to cope, something bigger is being missed.

That's when you need a professional assessment, not another prescription.

5. **Let your body do the work.** Always treat the medication as the assistant, not the leader. The medication can help you move, but only the movement can change the condition. Your body does the heavy lifting; the medication is simply there to back you up.

Now you have a plan: tablets for short-term relief, injections for short-term resets or smoothing movement, and strength for long-term change. You don't need to fear medication. You just need to use it the way it was meant to be used: as a window of opportunity, not the whole strategy. Once you see it that way, something important starts to shift.

The moment tablets stop controlling you

There's a point in recovery where you stop asking, 'Which tablet should I take?' and start asking, 'What does my body actually need?'

That's the real turning point. Tablets can dull pain, injections can calm irritation, but only you can rebuild the joint. Once you see that clearly, you stop feeling trapped by medication. You stop taking tablets just in case. You stop fearing the flare. You stop believing your body is too fragile to cope without a pill keeping you upright.

You start using medication on your terms. You start trusting movement again. You start feeling stronger week by week. You realise you've been capable all along; you just needed the right plan, not more medication.

This isn't about being drug-free. It's about being back in control. It's about knowing when medication helps and when it holds you back. The moment you lean back into your body instead of leaning on tablets, the whole story of your recovery begins to change. Drugs can open a window, but they can't move your body through it. That part is yours.

If Chapter 8 was about stepping out of the trap, the next chapter is about going forward.

9

Mindset – Why Your Mind Might Be Working Against You And How To Change It

Most people don't get stuck because of arthritis. They get stuck because of fear, and fear is learned, which means it can be unlearned.

This is where I need to rewind for a moment. Up to now, I've talked about how recovery starts with the body, because this is where most people expect it to begin, but in reality, it starts with the mind. I see it every day in clinic. Two people with the same problem, the same scan, the same diagnosis, yet one keeps moving and improves, while the other one tightens up, shuts down, and spirals.

The difference isn't in their joints. It's in their mindset.

Your thoughts can tighten your muscles faster than arthritis ever will. That's how fear works. One flare-up or sharp twinge, and suddenly your whole system goes into protection mode. Not because anything is damaged, but because your brain thinks it might be, and once that fear creeps in, your body moves differently. You take fewer steps, trust yourself less, and confidence slowly drains away. The trap isn't the pain; it's everything fear wraps around it.

Being a physio often means being a counsellor first. When people walk through my door, they're not worried about pain; they're worried about what the pain means. Does it mean their joints are wearing out? Does it mean their days of walking, travelling, or playing with their grandkids are numbered? Has something gone, slipped, or cracked? Nine times out of ten, the fear is louder than the symptoms.

Fear changes how you move. It tightens your muscles, stiffens your joints, and ramps up your nervous system. You can't rebuild strength on top of fear. You can't improve mobility when your whole body is acting like you're walking across broken glass. That's why this chapter matters so much: you have to address the mindset before anything else in this book really clicks.

I've seen Olympic athletes trust their bodies with a torn hamstring more than many people over fifty trust theirs after a simple arthritis flare-up. The injury isn't the difference – the mindset is. The athletes aren't braver or tougher; they've just learned how to interpret signals. They know the difference between discomfort and damage. Most people never get taught this, so every new ache feels threatening, and every flare feels like a setback.

A mindset isn't a personality trait; it's a skill. Like strength, mobility, or balance, it can be trained. You don't need to become positive or think happy thoughts; you simply need to understand what your body is trying to tell you, and how to stop your brain from jumping to the worst-case scenario every time something twinges.

Your body isn't fragile. It's conditioned, often by years of fear, stress, and worry, and conditioning can be undone. Every time you've walked off some stiffness or felt your back loosen after a few minutes of pottering around the house, you've experienced that shift. Your body responds when you give it a chance. This chapter will help you create more of those chances.

When life loads up, pain follows

Being a physio is often very different to what people imagine. Yes, I assess joints and muscles, but a large part of my job is simply listening, because once people start talking, the real story comes out.

I've had plenty of appointments where, within minutes, people open up about caring for a spouse, coping with grief, dealing with a house move, a family fallout, or just the sheer effort of keeping life together. Those conversations usually tell me far more about their pain than any scan ever could.

Often, your joints aren't the problem; your life load is.

Your nervous system doesn't distinguish between physical and emotional strain; it treats them as the same thing. When there's too much going on, the body reacts. You tighten up. Your breathing changes. Your sleep gets lighter. Your tolerance drops, and the little aches you'd usually ignore suddenly feel like something more serious. Most people blame arthritis, but the spark often comes from something else entirely.

This is why talking helps. When someone finally says, 'I've been under so much pressure recently,' their shoulders drop, their breathing eases, and the body follows. Often, the biggest relief comes not from treatment, but from finally realising the problem isn't their joints giving up; it's everything else piling on top.

That realisation alone changes everything. It stops the catastrophising, it calms the system, it reduces fear, and once the nervous system settles, movement starts to feel safe again. This is why mindset matters – not as a motivational slogan, but as a practical tool that changes how your body behaves.

If your life is overloaded with stress, responsibility, sleepless nights, and emotional weight, your pain will mirror it. Once you understand that relationship, you can finally start to influence it.

When pain becomes part of your role

Not every mindset trap shows up as fear or stress. Sometimes it comes from something far deeper: a shift in identity, a loss of purpose, or a life that has changed quicker than someone can adapt to. I saw this clearly with Jane, a woman in her late sixties who arrived in the clinic convinced she needed a knee replacement.

On the surface, her knee made no sense. Her strength was improving, and her movement was better. The exercises suited her. Nothing pointed towards a structural problem, yet week after week, nothing changed. The pain didn't budge. Every follow-up felt the same. She was doing everything right, but nothing was moving forward.

It wasn't until she started talking about her life that the real picture became obvious.

Jane's husband had died a year earlier, almost to the day. They had been together for decades, and his loss didn't just leave a gap in her home; it left a gap in her identity. She described the following months as 'walking around without a role', and it showed.

Her son lived hours away and was wrapped up with work and young kids. She didn't get on with her daughter-in-law, so visits were strained and rare. She hardly saw her grandchildren, as she never felt welcome enough to ask. Money was tight, and every week there seemed to be something else: the boiler service, the car's MOT, the house feeling too big. There was always something heavy sitting on her shoulders.

With all that going on, her pain had become the one constant. The thing she could point to that explained why life felt so hard. It slipped into how she spoke about herself, how she filled her days, how she justified slowing down. It wasn't just her knee anymore; it had woven itself into the space her husband used to occupy.

When we finally talked about this, properly, something changed. She realised she wasn't stuck because of her knee. She was stuck because she had nothing pulling her forward. No purpose, no routine, no sense of what life looked like without him. The knee pain had simply filled the void.

Once she saw that, the entire tone of our conversation shifted. Rehab became less about 'fixing the knee' and more about rebuilding a life with space for movement, connection, and small steps towards independence. Her body wasn't a barrier. The grief was.

This is one of the hardest mindset traps to spot because it has nothing to do with willpower or effort. It's about identity. When pain becomes part of who you are, it takes time, honesty, and the right support to untangle it, but once that work begins, the body often follows.

Your why

When someone sits down in front of me for the first time, I always ask the same question: 'What do you want to achieve from coming here?' Almost everyone gives me the same surface-level answer: 'I just want to be pain-free.'

Of course they do, it's the most obvious reason they're here. Nobody books physio because everything feels wonderful, but 'pain-free' is the safe response people give before they've had the chance to think deeper about what's really changed in their life.

I always follow up. Not to pressure anyone, but because the first answer is never the whole story. I ask slightly deeper questions like:

- What's the pain getting in the way of?
- What are you missing out on?
- If the pain vanished tomorrow, what would you go straight back to?

That's when people pause, because they're not just dealing with pain; they're dealing with things they've lost. They're missing the life they had before things tightened up, stiffened up, or slowed down. They're grieving the ease with which they once moved, the confidence they used to feel, and the independence they didn't realise they'd lost until it had already slipped away. They're grieving the version of themselves who didn't have to think about stairs, long walks, holidays, bending down, or getting out of a chair.

Once we gently explore that, the real reasons begin to surface.

Someone will tell me they can't get on the floor with their grandchildren anymore, or they avoid picking them up because they're frightened their joints will give way. Another will realise they've stopped going on holidays because the thought of long airport walks and hotel corridors feels overwhelming. Someone else admits they've stepped back from social plans because they don't like how stiff and old they look when they get up from a chair.

Then there are the examples that carry a different sort of weight. People who no longer enjoy hobbies or hardly see their friends. People who feel embarrassed to join their family on a walk because they know they'll be slow and don't want to hold everyone up. People who worry about becoming a burden, or who feel their world has quietly narrowed without anyone really noticing.

After more than twenty years of working with people over fifty, I can tell you this with absolute certainty: the turning point in recovery rarely comes from an exercise. It comes from understanding what pain has taken from your life.

It's rarely a big confession. It's the gradual losses that build over months and years, and once people say it out loud, I can almost see the shift. They stop talking about joints and start talking about life. About independence. About identity. About the everyday things that give structure and meaning to their days.

Pain-free isn't a goal. It's a hope. A *why* is what gets you moving again.

Before you read any further, I want you to do something important. Grab a pen. Write down what your pain is actually costing you, what you're missing out on, and what you're afraid of losing. One sentence or even a few words is enough.

Now stick it somewhere you'll see it every day. The fridge works well. Remind yourself of the life you want to get back to, and the parts of you that you're not ready to lose.

Your why doesn't have to impress anyone. It just has to be honest. When it is, it becomes the anchor that steadies you during the tough days – the days when you're stiff, tired, frustrated, or doubting the process – because at that point, you're not doing the work for a knee or a back. You're doing it for the life that sits in front of it.

Are you getting help from people you trust?

Once someone knows their why, the next question is whether they're getting help from someone they actually trust. It sounds simple, but it's one of the biggest turning points in recovery, because if you don't trust the person guiding you, you'll always second-guess their advice, hold back when you should push, and drift away when progress slows.

A lot of people, especially those over fifty, arrive at my clinic after months or sometimes years of feeling dismissed. They've been told it's just wear and tear or part of getting older, or they should 'take these tablets and see how you get on'. Ten-minute appointments, rushed explanations, vague reassurance, no plan. It's not the GP's fault; the system is under impossible pressure, but the result is the same. People leave appointments without clarity.

When you don't have clarity, you lose trust. When you lose trust, you lose confidence. When you lose confidence, you move less, and everything gets worse from there.

That is why physiotherapy is never just about joints and muscles. It's a relationship. A partnership. So much of what we do in clinic is simply explaining, reassuring, guiding, and giving people back a sense of control.

A process like this works best when both sides are clear, honest, and pulling in the same direction. When you feel heard, understood, and supported, something shifts. Your system settles. Your confidence grows. Movement feels less risky, and progress finally starts to happen.

Recovery isn't about doing everything perfectly; it's about working with someone you can trust enough to keep going. Things will get messy, confusing, or frustrating; they always do. That's where trust matters most. It's the thing that stops people from giving up just when they're about to turn a corner.

Trust flips the whole recovery game. It takes you out of fear mode and puts you back in control.

Managing stress, the enemy of repair

By the time someone walks into my clinic, stress isn't sitting quietly in the background anymore. It's running the show. Not the dramatic, life-falling-apart kind of stress people imagine, but the slow, steady strain that builds when you're looking after a partner, trying to keep work and family afloat, worrying about money, or dealing with loss. It sits in the background, chips away at you, and half the time you don't even realise how much it's taken out of you.

Stress changes how your body feels long before anything changes in your joints. When you're stressed, worried, or overwhelmed, your nervous system goes on high alert. It starts looking for danger everywhere, and when your brain is on edge like that, your body follows. You tense up. You hold your breath. You move as if you're expecting something to hurt, even when nothing's actually happened yet.

There are brain scan studies that prove this.[72] People under stress light up threat and pain areas in the brain before they even move. In some cases, just watching someone else bend or twist is enough to set it off. That's why stress makes everything feel worse, not because the joint has suddenly changed, but because your nervous system has.

This is exactly why people tell me their pain has come out of nowhere, but when we talk it through, it rarely comes out of nowhere at all. It comes from a period of life where they've been trying to hold everything together. They haven't had a moment to breathe, never mind recover. Their system has been locked in alert mode for so long that the body starts behaving as though even normal movement needs protecting.

Stress doesn't have to cause pain to make it worse; it simply lowers the threshold at which things feel uncomfortable. It tightens muscles, it shortens movement, it changes posture, and it keeps you in a guarded state. Guarded bodies struggle to move freely, which is why a small ache on a calm week can feel like a major setback during a stressful one.

Stress doesn't just influence how pain feels; it shapes what you do in response to it. When life feels overwhelming, it's no surprise that you pull back. You move less, you skip walks because you're tired, and you miss the exercises you're meant to do. When your head's full, everything feels heavier than it should. The stiffness doesn't get challenged, so it hangs around, and the less you do, the more your confidence slips. It's a cycle, not a flaw.

This is why managing stress isn't a luxury; it's a key part of getting your confidence back. You don't need meditation apps, retreats, or perfect routines. You simply need moments in the day when your system can settle, instead of constantly being dragged forward by life. That might be ten minutes with a coffee before the house wakes up, a gentle walk after dinner, five minutes of slow breathing at the end of the day, or just giving yourself permission to say no to things you don't have capacity for.

When stress reduces even slightly, the whole body becomes less reactive. Movements feel safer, flares feel smaller, you stop bracing as much and assuming the worst. Then the exercises you're already doing begin to land properly because your system isn't fighting against you.

You don't need a stress-free life to make progress; nobody has that. You just need enough calm in the system for your body to stop feeling under threat. Once that happens, everything else becomes easier.

Relationships, community, and your support network

When we talk about mindset, most people assume we're talking about motivation, positivity, or mental toughness, but recovery has far less to do with willpower and far more to do with the people you're surrounded by. Your support network, or lack of one, has a massive influence on how you behave, how confident you feel, and how quickly you make progress. I see it all the time.

Some people move forward because they've got someone in their corner: someone who listens, encourages them, and gives them a nudge on the days they'd otherwise let things slide. Others struggle, not because their joints are worse, but because they're carrying everything on their own or surrounded by people who unintentionally fuel their fear.

It's common for someone to say, 'My wife/husband keeps telling me not to push it just in case something goes wrong.' It's said with love, but another person's worry becomes your worry. You move more cautiously, you avoid testing yourself, you take fewer chances, and your confidence shrinks.

Then there are people with someone beside them saying, 'You're doing well, keep going.' I see the difference immediately. They stand a little taller. They take ownership. They try again after a setback. Support doesn't remove pain, but it completely changes how you respond to it.

There's another layer to this that people don't talk about. Many over-fifties are in caring roles, looking after their spouse, supporting elderly parents, helping with grandchildren, and juggling work and family. They spend their days meeting everybody else's needs, and their own health slips further and further down the list. By the time they sit in front of me, they're exhausted. Not necessarily physically, but emotionally, and when you're emotionally drained, you simply don't have the energy to invest in yourself.

It's not selfish to prioritise your own recovery; it's necessary. You can't pour from an empty cup, and you can't rebuild strength and confidence when every ounce of your energy is spent on everyone else. I've lost count of the number of times someone has said, 'I feel guilty taking time for myself,' as if looking after their joints and mobility is a luxury rather than a basic requirement for a healthy life.

A strong support network isn't just about encouragement. It's about space – space to look after yourself, space to rest, space to follow through on the work you do with your physiotherapist in the clinic. It's about having people around you who understand that your progress depends on consistency and patience, not panic.

If you don't have that network right now, it doesn't mean you can't recover. It simply means you need to be more intentional about the influences you allow in. Choose to spend time with people who move, who think proactively, who talk about possibilities rather than limitations. Choose people who make you feel capable, not fragile.

You only have to look at places in the world where people stay active well into their eighties and nineties to see the power of community in action. Okinawa, a region of Japan often studied for longevity, is a good example.[73] Daily life there is naturally active. People walk, garden, dance, chat with neighbours, take part in small rituals, and stay connected to groups they've belonged to for decades. Researchers studying these long-living populations point to the same pattern again and again: it's the combination of constant low-level movement and strong social ties that keeps people mobile.

Large studies support the same pattern. Older adults who have stronger social networks don't just feel better emotionally than those who don't; they actually have better strength, balance, and mobility, and are far less likely to lose independence later in life.[74]

Most people in their fifties, sixties, and seventies know this instinctively. They'll tell me, 'I used to be better when I was busy,' or 'I walked more when I had people to walk with,' or 'I kept up with things when I was part of a group.' It's rarely the pain that takes people away from activity; it's losing the environment that made activity feel normal.

I see this in the clinic all the time. Someone will stop playing walking football after an injury, and without that group around them, their activity levels collapse. Another person will drift away from a walking club or the church community and gradually lose the routine that once kept them mobile and socially connected. Pain doesn't remove those habits; isolation does.

Being around people who move makes you more likely to move, and the opposite is true as well. If you spend most of your time with people who are inactive, fearful, negative about their health, or constantly reinforcing the idea that everything's getting worse with age, it's almost impossible not to absorb some of that mindset yourself. Being around people who talk positively about ageing makes you less frightened of it. Being around people who laugh, chat, and share the load makes everything feel lighter.

I'm not necessarily advocating joining a gym or signing up for something formal. It's about putting yourself in environments where movement happens naturally. For some, that's swimming or paddle tennis. For others, it's a weekly dance class, a Tai Chi group, a gardening project, a book club, a church group, or simply a few friends who meet for regular walks.

If your world has become smaller over the years through pain, bereavement, caring responsibilities, or simple drift, one of the most powerful things you can do for your recovery is gently rebuild some form of community around you. Movement sticks better when it has company.

Mindset drives behaviour

By now, you can probably see that pain isn't just a physical experience; it's shaped by everything around it. Your thoughts, your fears, your relationships, your stress levels, your sense of purpose, your routines, your losses, your community – they all influence how your body behaves long before you ever lift a weight or stretch a muscle.

When people feel stuck, it's rarely because their joints are beyond help. More often, it's because their mindset has been pulled into a place where movement feels threatening, confidence feels fragile, and life has become a little too small. Pain thrives in that space. It grows in isolation, in fear and uncertainty, and in the stories we tell ourselves about what our bodies can and can't do.

The opposite is also true. When someone understands what's really driving their pain, when they reconnect with their why, when they feel supported, when they're part of a community that values movement, something shifts. The nervous system settles, their confidence returns, their decisions change; and once behaviour changes, the body follows.

This is why mindset sits at the front of recovery. You can have the perfect exercise plan on paper, but if your mind is stuck in threat mode, worried, overwhelmed, or expecting the worst, your body pushes back. It guards. It tightens. It resists.

When your mind feels safer, and you're clear on what you're trying to achieve, the whole system becomes more willing to move. Everything feels a little less risky.

The people who do best in middle age and beyond aren't the ones with the strongest muscles; they're the ones who change the way they read their symptoms. They stop jumping to catastrophic conclusions. They set meaningful goals. They keep themselves moving on the days they don't feel perfect. They surround themselves with people and environments that make progress feel possible instead of frightening.

Mindset isn't about pretending everything is fine. It's not about ignoring pain or forcing positivity. It's about understanding your body well enough that you can make decisions from clarity rather than fear.

When that shift happens, even the small things have an impact: a short walk, a few minutes of strength work, a simple routine you stick to. These aren't just exercises; they are behaviours that tell your nervous system, 'I'm safe, I'm capable, I can do this.' Over time, this message becomes stronger than the pain.

You don't need to fix everything at once; you just need to create the kind of environment, inside your mind and around your life, where recovery has a chance to take hold. Once it does, it's remarkable how quickly things change.

Pain shrinks the world. Mindset expands it again. It just needs the right support, which is why the next chapter looks at tools that improve healing, support recovery, calm the nervous system, and make movement feel easier again.

10
Technology Behind Recovery

Athletes don't bounce back from injury because they're special. They bounce back because they use technology that most people over fifty don't have access to.

At least, this used to be the case. Now modern tools are no longer just for elite athletes. More technology than ever is available through private physio practices. I've written this chapter to get you up to speed.

For years, advanced recovery tools lived in a completely different world: the world of elite athletes, Premier League medical rooms, Olympic rehab centres, and celebrity headlines. Many people still picture hyperbaric oxygen as the thing that Michael Jackson supposedly slept in to stay young. It turned out to be a PR stunt, apparently, but it's imprinted on children of the eighties.

Many, including myself, remember the photos of David Beckham in 2002 and Wayne Rooney in 2006, both sitting inside a hyperbaric oxygen chamber trying to heal broken metatarsals in time for the World Cup. Back then, it looked almost sci-fi, something reserved for global superstars with million-pound careers on the line. For them, the speed of recovery wasn't a luxury. It was everything.

While I worked with elite athletes, I saw it first-hand. When their joints hurt or something tightened, they didn't just stretch and hope. They used science-backed recovery protocols, including hyperbaric oxygen therapy, red light therapy, neuromuscular stimulation, sleep tracking, and data monitoring, long before the public ever heard of them.

Red light therapy? Most people think of beauty salons or those LED face masks celebrities use to look younger. In elite sport, it's been cutting-edge recovery technology for years.

Neurostimulation? Most people picture a basic transcutaneous electrical nerve stimulation (TENS) machine. What athletes use is on a completely different level.

What's changed is this: the tools aren't elite anymore. They're accessible, researched, and helping ordinary people move better than they have in years.

To prove the point, I'm writing this section inside a hyperbaric chamber. No entourage. No Hollywood budget. The same physiological benefits Beckham and Rooney were chasing – benefits I now use myself for recovery, clarity, and long-term health – are helping ordinary people improve how they feel and how they move.

Technology isn't a shortcut; it's an advantage, a way of creating the same recovery environment athletes get without needing to be one. These tools don't replace movement, strength, or mindset; nothing does, but they do change the speed, ease, and consistency of your results. Elite recovery works because the environment works, and now that environment is finally accessible.

Collecting data: The sports scientist on your wrist

Before we get into hyperbaric oxygen, red light therapy, or Neubie technology, we need to talk about something far simpler: the tools you likely already own, but barely use. Elite recovery never started with fancy machines. It started with measuring what the body was doing.

When I worked with athletes, nothing was left to chance. Their sleep, effort, recovery, stress, and workload were monitored every day. Not to be clever, but because guessing leads to injury, and clarity leads to progress and performance. Movement, strength, and rehab all landed better when the data lined up with the plan.

Most people over fifty already have access to the same kind of information, usually sitting on their wrist, but instead of treating their smart watch like a sports scientist, they use it like a clock. This is one of the biggest differences between athletes and the average person. Athletes know what their body is doing before their body tells them. Most people wait until their joints are shouting, and by the time their body shouts, they're already behind.

Take sleep. When an athlete's sleep dips, their recovery slows, performance drops, and their joints feel heavy the next day. They adjust because they can see it happening in black and white. Most people don't notice the link; they just wake stiff, assume it's arthritis, and miss the real reason entirely: their body is under-recovered, not broken.

Alternatively, look at heart rate. A rising resting heart rate is often a sign of stress, fatigue, or illness before symptoms appear. Athletes have used this for years to avoid overtraining and wiping themselves out. Most people only notice something's wrong when their back or knee starts moaning, and by then it's too late to avoid a flare.

Then there's heart rate variability (HRV) – the fluctuation in the time between your heartbeats. Think of it as a rough indicator of how well your body is coping with whatever life is throwing at you and how much capacity it has left in the tank. Athletes use HRV to know when to push and when to back off, and people over fifty can use it in exactly the same way.

You don't need to be an athlete for it to make sense. If the HRV number dips, it usually means your system is under load. Poor sleep, stress, illness, pain, or a flare-up will often push it down. That's your cue to give yourself a bit more margin that day. Walk instead of push. Maintain rather than build. When HRV is higher, it generally means your body is coping well. You've got more room to do a bit extra without tipping things over.

There isn't a 'good' number you need to hit. What matters is your pattern. Your low days. Your higher days. Used well, HRV helps you avoid walking straight into flare-ups. Used badly, it becomes another thing to worry about, so be careful not to drown in the data. If it ramps up your anxiety, the tool has become a problem.

You don't need spreadsheets or weekly reports breathing down your neck. You just need awareness, because once you see a pattern, for example 'On the days I sleep badly, my back is worse,' the shift is simple. The feedback changes your decisions.

I see it every week in clinic. Someone sits in front of me with an expensive smart watch on their wrist and says, 'I'm so stiff in the mornings.' When we open the sleep data, it's there in black and white: three nights of broken sleep, then a flare-up.

A simple walking programme, a gentle running progression like Couch to 5K, or a runner's app that breaks things into clear, manageable steps – these give you structure, routine, and accountability, which are all things people tell me they struggle with after fifty. They tell me they just need something to follow. Athletes have physios and coaches. You have apps. The principle is the same: it's easier to follow a clear plan than to wing it.

Here's why this section comes before we look in detail at hyperbaric oxygen, red light therapy, and the Neubie: elite tools work best on a body that already has the basics in place. Good sleep. A bit of movement. Less background stress. A clearer picture of what your body is doing day to day.

Technology doesn't replace those things; it amplifies them. That's why athletes used these tools long before the public did, and it's why people over fifty benefit most when they use technology to support the foundations, not dodge them.

When you understand your patterns, your body becomes easy to help. Once your body is easy to help, the advanced tools make a lot more sense.

Before we examine those advanced tools, let's have a look at some popular trends in recovery options. What helps, what doesn't, and what should you stop wasting your money on?

Recovery tools

Walk into any gym, scroll through social media, or watch daytime TV, and you'll see the same thing: a conveyor belt of recovery gadgets, miracle devices, and 'must-have' tools that promise to take your pain away.

Recovery tools are supposed to make movement easier, not confuse you or empty your bank account. Let me save you some time, money, and frustration, cut through the marketing, and talk about what actually works for people over fifty with joint stiffness and arthritis. Most of it is noise. Some of it helps. A small handful of these tools are actually worth using – but only if you understand what they really do. I've given each a rating based on its usefulness.

Ice baths

Everyone is plunging into freezing tubs at the moment. It looks heroic. It feels extreme. It's the trend social media loves, but your joints might not.

Athletes don't use ice baths for arthritis. They use them to survive brutal training loads. Cold plunges can reduce general muscle soreness, and they can give you a short-term energy kick, but for arthritic joints? Cold often makes stiffness worse, not better. If you enjoy the shock and feel great afterwards, fine, but don't kid yourself that an ice bath is doing anything meaningful for your hips or knees.

Rating: Optional. Not essential. Not joint-specific.

Saunas

More helpful for stiff or arthritic joints, but still not a fix, saunas sit on the opposite end of the spectrum to ice baths. The heat relaxes tight muscles, improves circulation, calms your nervous system, and improves sleep, which matters for arthritis. There's even research linking regular sauna use with better cardiovascular health and lower stress – great for recovery in general.[75]

Then again, a sauna will not repair cartilage, it will not replace strength work, and it definitely won't fix years of stiffness on its own. If you tolerate heat well and enjoy the routine, it's a solid add-on. If you walk out feeling dizzy, flushed, or drained, skip it.

Rating: Helpful support tool. Not treatment.

Cryotherapy

With their three minutes of freezing silence, cryotherapy chambers look impressive. They make great Instagram content. They suggest you are doing something extreme for your health, but do they help arthritis?

No.

Cryotherapy gives a quick endorphin lift, temporary soreness reduction, and a mental reset feeling. That's about it. It doesn't improve mobility. It doesn't reduce arthritic stiffness. It doesn't produce long-term relief. Most professional athletes use it for mood, not joints, and for many people over fifty, the extreme cold tightens joints once the initial buzz wears off.

Rating: Fun for some, pointless for most. Not a joint tool.

Massage guns

Great warm-up, but a terrible long-term plan, massage guns are everywhere now. Yes, I use them in clinic, but let's be honest about what they do.

They loosen tight muscles, they make exercises easier to get into, and they help you move with more confidence. That's it. They do not fix muscle imbalances, strengthen weak glutes, change the way a joint loads, or replace structured rehab.

Here's how to employ a massage gun properly: use it to get moving. Don't rely on it to keep you moving.

Rating: Useful warm-up tool. Not a solution.

TENS machine

People love the electrical stimulation that comes from TENS machines because it makes them feel like they're doing something. Yes, TENS can reduce the perception of pain. It can distract a sensitive nervous system. It can help you tolerate movement, but let's not overstate it.

TENS is relief without progress. It does nothing to change the cause of the problem. If you use the relief to walk more, stretch better, or strengthen properly, great. If you use it to sit more comfortably while nothing else changes, all you've done is make sitting easier.

Rating: Fine if it leads to movement. Pointless if it replaces it.

Compression boots and recovery pants

You've probably seen these: big inflatable boots or trousers that squeeze your legs rhythmically. They're fantastic for athletes between games or events. They help with circulation, they make heavy legs feel lighter, but if you think they'll fix your knee arthritis, you're being sold a dream. Walking, calf strength, and structured pacing do far more for joint health than any pair of expensive air-filled trousers.

Rating: Luxury item. Impressive, but not essential. Not required for progress.

Home cardio and gym equipment

Here's a familiar story. Someone buys a treadmill. They use it three times. It becomes a coat stand. It's not the treadmill that's failed; it's the habit.

If you know you'll use it consistently, a home gym is brilliant. It gives you options and keeps you moving in bad weather. If you're buying out of guilt or desperation rather than because you know exactly how you'll use it, that's your warning sign. Save your money. Start with walking, bodyweight strength work, and routine. Earn your equipment.

Rating: High value if used. High regret if not.

What should you actually do with all this?

Let's strip it right back. No tool replaces movement, strength, sleep, stress management, and pacing. It only makes things easier. If a tool helps you move better tomorrow, great, use it. If it doesn't, it's clutter.

As long as these everyday tools support your foundations, advanced technologies can work the way they should. Most people skip the basics and jump straight to expensive kit. That's why they get poor results. Build the foundations first. Then layer on the advanced tools. That's how athletes recover fast, and it's how you will make the biggest difference to your joints.

Now let's look at the first advanced tool, the one that changes the recovery environment itself.

Hyperbaric oxygen therapy (HBOT)

Your recovery isn't slow because of age. It's slow because your body is low on oxygen.

Arthritis doesn't just make joints ache; it slows everything around them. Recovery drags, mornings feel heavier, and muscles fatigue sooner than they should. You can sleep well and still wake up feeling like you're already behind. This isn't ageing. It's a system running without enough oxygen to do its job properly. It's like running a house on half its electricity. Everything still works, just not well, and never at the speed you need it to.

HBOT changes that. Inside the chamber, the pressure rises, and your body takes in a flood of oxygen far beyond what's possible in ordinary breathing. You'll feel a pressure similar to when you're on a plane; your ears may pop, but your body knows exactly what to do. That oxygen dissolves into your plasma as well as your red blood cells, which means it can reach stiff, irritated, slow-healing tissues that don't normally get much oxygen at all. If arthritis is a long-lasting traffic jam, HBOT is the moment the roads clear and the repair crews can finally get through.

It isn't a quick fix, and it's not supposed to be. Chronic problems don't respond to one-off attempts. HBOT works the same way strength does: small, repeated doses that build momentum. The early changes are subtle: better sleep, less morning stiffness, clearer thinking. These changes matter. They show inflammation is settling and your system is finally getting the oxygen it needs.

The deeper shift comes later. Most people notice real changes somewhere between ten and twenty sessions. Not because the chamber becomes stronger, but because chronic inflammation needs repeated oxygen exposure. It's cumulative. Each session adds to the last, and your body slowly starts to behave differently.

Oxygen plays a far bigger role in easing arthritis than most people realise. When a joint is irritated, everything around it has to work harder. The muscles tighten to protect it. The nervous system keeps everything on high alert. All of that takes energy, but as you get older, you naturally deliver a bit less oxygen to those same tissues. You've got a joint that needs more and a system that's giving less. It's no wonder things feel slow, heavy, or constantly on the edge of a flare.

HBOT helps close that gap. That's why people often describe feeling lighter or less inflamed, not because anything dramatic happens in one session, but because the body finally stops fighting itself all day.

I use HBOT for similar reasons. I'm not injured. I use it to keep my head sharp, recover quicker after training, and stop the fatigue that builds slowly between busy clinic days. I'll be honest: when I'm consistently using it, it feels like I'm cheating. Everything just works better.

Give the cells what they need and they behave better. When they behave better, you feel better. HBOT doesn't fix arthritis, but it gives the system the oxygen it hasn't had for years. When the system improves, everything else – movement, strength, confidence – has room to improve with it.

Once the system has the oxygen it needs, the next step is calming the irritated tissues themselves. That's where red light therapy comes in.

Red light therapy

Arthritis doesn't just affect the joint. It irritates everything around it. The tissues stay warm, swollen, and sensitive. Muscles tighten. The whole area becomes reactive as it's stuck halfway between tension and inflammation.

Red light therapy turns that irritation down, helping stiff, irritated joints behave better. It uses specific wavelengths of light, the same range your cells naturally respond to, to boost how well they produce energy. Think of it as giving tired tissues a power source they've been running low on for years. When cells have more energy available, they repair faster, settle inflammation sooner, and stop behaving like they're under threat all the time. That's why joints often feel looser, lighter, and less angry afterwards. You haven't changed your arthritis; you've changed the environment it sits in.

If HBOT, with its injection of oxygen, clears the road so repair crews can get through, red light improves the road surface itself by reducing irritation. The tissues become less irritable, less swollen, and more willing to move. The joint doesn't feel as guarded because the tissue around it isn't constantly shouting.

You'll usually notice small but important changes first: easier bending, less morning stiffness, a joint that doesn't bite the moment you load it. These early shifts matter. They make strength work easier, they reduce flare-ups, and they give you more confidence to move, which is exactly what most people with arthritis need.

The research is catching up with what I see in clinic. Studies show improvements in pain, inflammation, joint stiffness, and general function when red light is used consistently.[76] None of this is magic. It's simply energy helping irritated tissues behave like healthy tissues again.

Like HBOT, red light won't reverse arthritis, but it calms the irritated tissues that make it feel worse. When the irritation settles, the joint becomes easier to work with.

Once the tissues are calmer, the next step is teaching your muscles how to move properly again with Neubie electrical stimulation therapy.

Neubie therapy

Arthritis doesn't just irritate joints. It changes how your muscles behave. You've seen this already in earlier chapters: when something hurts, your system tightens around it, muscles switch off, others overwork, and your movement becomes guarded and smaller. Over time, these patterns become habits. Not because you're weak, but because your nervous system is protecting you.

Neubie helps undo that, teaching your muscles to work properly again. It uses a specific form of direct current electrical stimulation that taps into your nervous system and reconnects the brain's messages to activate your muscles. This identifies which muscles are actually doing their job and which ones have quietly dropped out.

Most people are shocked by what we find. A muscle they thought was strong starts to shake the moment we test it. One that feels tight is actually doing the work for three others that aren't firing at all. This isn't failure, it's information. It tells us exactly where muscles' movement has been compensating.

Think of Neubie like switching a tripped fuse back on. The power was always there; it just wasn't getting through. Once the signal returns, the muscle wakes up and movement feels cleaner again.

What people notice first is control. A knee that wobbled is suddenly steadier. A hip that dragged feels awake again. Steps are more confident. Exercises stop feeling like guesswork. This matters with arthritis. When the muscles fire at the right time, the joint feels protected and safe rather than threatened, and when that happens, stiffness reduces, strength work actually sticks, and flare-ups become far less common.

Neubie gives immediate feedback through how the muscles respond, so we can train them under load without guessing. Too much activation? It shows up straight away. Not enough? Neubie shows that too. You learn how to move without the compensations your body has been hiding behind. For many people, it's the first time they've felt a muscle work the way it's supposed to in years.

The early research on neuromuscular electrical stimulation, the same principle used by devices like Neubie, mirrors what I see in clinic.[77] Neubie can often strengthen an irritated joint without even moving it. The muscle works hard, the joint stays calm: the perfect combination for arthritis. It reduces guarding and protective tension, which immediately makes movement easier.

People recovering from major injuries regain strength, mobility, and confidence much faster when Neubie is added to their rehab. A recent knee replacement case study shared by NeuFit showed faster pain reduction, earlier return of quadriceps strength, and quicker progress to functional mobility when Neubie was used alongside exercise.[78]

Many cases use all three technologies. A few months ago, in clinic, I worked with a man in his early sixties, David, who'd just had a hip replacement. He was doing everything right, but his recovery felt painfully slow. His wound was healing, but the swelling lingered. His hip stayed warm most days, and any time he tried to move on with his exercises, he hit the same wall of stiffness and irritation.

We started with the Neubie straight away. After a hip replacement, it's very common for the key muscles to switch off; they've literally been cut through during surgery, so the nervous system shuts them down to protect them. Even though his joint wasn't ready for traditional strengthening, those muscles still needed waking up. Neubie is perfect for that stage. It let us load the muscles without putting any stress through the new joint.

Within minutes, it was obvious which muscles had switched off and which ones were doing all the guarding. The ones meant to support his hip were barely firing; the surrounding tissues were working overtime to keep him safe.

At the same time, we introduced HBOT. A hip replacement creates a huge oxygen demand: the tissue has been cut, moved, stitched, and asked to repair at speed. HBOT is brilliant for that. It floods the area with the oxygen the body needs for wound healing and calming inflammation. Within a week, he noticed the swelling easing. His sleep improved and his leg didn't feel as heavy.

However, the tissues were still irritable. The wound was closed and healing well, which meant we could safely add red light therapy to help the irritated tissues settle. The change was small but important: the hip felt less angry, movement became easier, and he could get into positions that had been too sharply painful or too tight a few days earlier.

Once the irritation had settled, the difference in his strength work was night and day. The muscles that had gone missing after surgery finally started showing up again. Movements that used to wobble were suddenly solid. Within a couple of weeks, his walking, which had been short and stiff, looked a lot more like it should've been from the start.

To be clear, it wasn't one miracle tool that did this. It was the combination that changed everything. HBOT and red light calmed the inflammation and sped up healing. Neubie rebuilt the muscle control that protects the joint.

None of it replaced his rehab; it simply removed the things that were slowing it. Once those barriers were out of the way, his progress moved quicker than either of us expected. He felt like he was finally getting somewhere instead of circling the same problems every week.

Some people use all three of these advanced tools. Some use one. Some use none. All that matters is whether they help you move better tomorrow than you do today, which has been the focus of the entire book. Physio at over fifty is about giving you hope. There's no inevitable entirely downward spiral. Movement can, and does, improve, no matter your age.

Conclusion: A Moment Of Clarity

This book was never about chasing pain away. It is about something deeper than that.

Most people I meet haven't failed to look after themselves. They've tried to do the right thing, resting when told to rest, stretching when told to stretch, taking the tablets they were prescribed, going for the scans they were sent for, and still been left unsure what any of it actually means.

They've rarely been given clarity. Without it, you start guessing. Pain gets mistaken for damage. Stiffness means decline. Getting older feels like your world is shrinking.

Those assumptions slowly change how you move, how you load your body, and how much trust you place in it. Over time, that does far more harm than arthritis ever could. That's not ageing. That's misunderstanding with consequences.

It is why I wrote this book.

I wrote it because I see the same pattern play out in the clinic every week. People aren't broken. They're out of shape, lacking strength, poorly informed, and understandably cautious after years of mixed messages. Once someone believes their body is fragile, they start behaving as if it is. Movement reduces. Confidence drops. Strength fades. Pain fills the space that is left behind.

When you change the story, your behaviour changes. When behaviour changes, your body responds even later in life. I've seen it too many times to ignore.

Throughout this book, we stripped things back to first principles. No trends, hacks, gimmicks, or miracle fixes. Just how the body works, how it adapts, and how it responds to the demands you place on it, or don't.

You've seen that joints don't do well being wrapped in cotton wool. Pain is not a reliable measure of damage. Rest can be useful, but only briefly. Strength, movement, sleep, and consistency matter far more than any single treatment. None of that is revolutionary. It's just been forgotten.

One of the most damaging ideas people carry into later life is the belief that improvement should be dramatic. Big breakthroughs. Sudden relief. A clear before and after.

Real progress after fifty is usually quiet and often slower than people expect. Morning routines don't take as long. Confidence returns without you noticing. Strength holds instead of fades.

It's walking the golf course without counting down the holes. Getting onto the floor with your grandchildren and back up again without planning the exit. Saying yes to things without first wondering how your joints will cope. It's doing everyday things without that constant background worry about becoming reliant on the people you care about. Flare-ups that settle quicker than they used to. A body you stop monitoring every five minutes.

I often see the moment things start to change. Someone stands up from the chair without thinking, then pauses and looks surprised. 'That felt easier,' they say. Nothing dramatic has happened. Their body has just begun to trust itself again.

Some people will feel better quickly. Others will need longer. Neither means you're doing it wrong. The goal was never perfection. The goal is resilience.

We've discussed pills clearly. Medication can be useful, especially during flares or when pain is getting in the way of movement and sleep. Used with a plan, it can buy you breathing space. Used without one, it often keeps the cycle going.

Tablets don't rebuild strength and they don't restore confidence, but when they help you move, train, and recover more consistently, they can be part of a sensible strategy rather than the whole strategy.

You also now have a better understanding of what helps and what makes things worse. You know which habits calm inflammation rather than fuel it, how food and recovery support your joints instead of sabotaging them, and how to spot the difference between useful discomfort and warning signs. That doesn't mean getting it perfect. It means making fewer panicked decisions and far more sensible ones. If this book has done its job, you'll now see your body less as something that's wearing out and more as something that adapts slowly, predictably, and in response to what you ask of it.

For some people, surgery may still become part of the story, and that isn't failure. What matters is that it's a considered decision, not one driven by fear or poor preparation. The stronger, fitter, and more confident you are beforehand, the better the surgery tends to go. Your recovery is faster, outcomes are more predictable, and you return to doing the things that matter to you sooner.

In that sense, everything you've read in this book applies whether surgery is on the horizon or not. That shift in perspective alone can change how you move, how you train, and how much confidence you carry back into everyday life.

Confidence matters, but not the kind that comes from gritting your teeth and pushing through pain. It's the confidence that comes from understanding what's happening in your body and knowing how to respond sensibly when things flare.

You don't need to overhaul everything at once. You don't need perfect days and you don't need to get it right all the time. What matters is getting started. Waiting for the perfect moment, or for pain to disappear completely, is still a decision, and it often keeps people stuck. You just need to keep the handbrake off long enough for momentum to build.

If you've taken anything from this book, let it be this: your body is not finished and your future is not fixed. There will always be setbacks. There will be days when things feel stiff, sore, or frustrating. That's not failure, that's biology. What matters is that you now have a framework for making sense of those moments rather than fearing them. You are no longer guessing, you are no longer waiting for permission, you are no longer assuming the worst, and that changes everything.

If you want more clarity

Some readers will close this book feeling confident enough to crack on. Others will feel reassured, but still unsure where to start or what matters most for their body. Both responses are completely normal.

If you're still unsure where to start, there's an optional online questionnaire that helps you step back, look at where you are right now, and decide what's worth focusing on first. You don't have to use it. It's there if you want a bit more clarity. You can access the questionnaire by visiting quiz.philthephysio.com/start-here or by scanning the QR code below:

Wherever you are right now, you're not too late. You haven't missed your chance. You've simply reached the point where understanding replaces fear, and that's where real progress begins. You don't need to wait for things to magically improve. You don't need to be braver or tougher. You just need to use what you now understand.

Your body isn't fragile. It's responsive. Once you stop treating it like it's finished, it behaves differently.

You're not guessing anymore. You know what helps. You know what holds you back. You know how to respond when things flare instead of panicking.

That's the shift.

From here on, you don't need perfect days or constant motivation. You don't need to fix everything at once. You just need to keep doing the things you now understand, often enough for your body to trust you again.

That's where strength comes back. Confidence follows and life stops slowly shrinking in the background.

Don't wait for pain to disappear before you act. Don't overthink the next step.

Use what you've learned. Stay sensible. Keep moving.

You've got this.

Notes

1 NICE, 'Chronic pain (primary and secondary) in over 16s: Assessment of all chronic pain and management of chronic primary pain', NICE Guideline NG193 (7 April 2021), www.nice.org.uk/guidance/ng193/chapter/recommendations, accessed 5 February 2026
2 S Tarannum, J Widdifield et al, 'Understanding sex-related differences in healthcare utilisation among patients: a population based study', *BMJ Journals*, 82:2, (16 September 2022), https://ard.bmj.com/content/82/2/283.info, accessed 11 Feb 2026
3 M Azzuan Ahmed, A Yusof et al, 'Effects of self-management program as adjunctive to usual rehabilitation exercise on pain and functional outcomes in knee osteoarthritis: A randomized controlled trial', National Library of Medicine, *JRHS*, 23:1 (30 March 2023), https://pmc.ncbi.nlm.nih.gov/articles/PMC10422143, accessed 11 February 2026
4 M Pahor, J M Guralnik et al, 'Effect of structured physical activity on prevention of major mobility disability in older adults', *JAMA Network*, 311:23 (18 June 2014), https://jamanetwork.com/journals/jama/fullarticle/1875328, accessed 11 February 2026

5 E Lunt, T Ong et al, 'The clinical usefulness of muscle mass and strength measures in older people: a systematic review', *Age and Ageing*, 50:1, 88–95 (January 2021), https://academic.oup.com/ageing/article/50/1/88/5872072, accessed 11 February 2026

6 NA Segal, NA Glass et al, 'Quadriceps weakness predicts risk for knee joint space narrowing in women in the MOST cohort', *Osteoarthritis and Cartilage*, 18:6, 769–75 (June 2010), https://doi.org/10.1016/j.joca.2010.02.002

7 AC da Silva, V Mapa et al, 'Progressive strength training can reverse sarcopenia stage in middle-aged and older adults regardless of their genetic profile', *Archives of Gerontology and Geriatrics* (7 September 2023), https://doi.org/10.1016/j.archger.2023.105182

8 AE Paluch, S Bajpai et al, 'Daily steps and all-cause mortality: a meta-analysis of 15 international cohorts', *The Lancet*, 7 (March 2002), www.thelancet.com/action/showPdf?pii=S2468-2667%2821%2900302-9, accessed 11 February 2026

9 M Mosley, 'Forget walking 10,000 steps a day' (BBC News, 31 January 2018), www.bbc.co.uk/news/health-42864061, accessed 11 February 2026

10 M Banach, J Lewek et al, 'The association between daily step count and all-cause and cardiovascular mortality: a meta-analysis', *EAPC*, 30:18, 1975–1985 (December 2023), https://doi.org/10.1093/eurjpc/zwad229, accessed 11 February 2026

11 A Mehdipour, S Malouka et al, 'Measurement properties of the usual and fast gait speed tests in community-dwelling older adults: a COSMIN-based systematic review', *Age and Ageing*, 53:3 (21 March 2024), https://pmc.ncbi.nlm.nih.gov/articles/PMC10958613, accessed 11 February 2026

12 AM Ramos, PJ M-Pardo et al, 'Resistance circuit training or walking training: Which program improves muscle strength and functional autonomy more in older women?', *International Journal of Environmental Research and Public Health* 19:14 (20 Jul 2022), https://pmc.ncbi.nlm.nih.gov/articles/PMC9319797, accessed 11 February 2026

13 Arthritis UK Homepage, www.arthritis-uk.org/information-and-support/understanding-arthritis/conditions/rheumatoid-arthritis, accessed 11 February 2026

14 S Tancer, BI Wallace, 'Advances in the Medical Treatment of Rheumatoid Arthritis', *Hand Clinics*, 41:1 (February 2025),

https://pmc.ncbi.nlm.nih.gov/articles/PMC12158440, accessed 11 February 2026

15 RF van Vollenhoven, 'Sex differences in rheumatoid arthritis: more than meets the eye…', *BMC Medicine*, 7:12 (30 March 2009), https://pmc.ncbi.nlm.nih.gov/articles/PMC2670321, accessed 11 February 2026

16 R Zhang and J Qu, 'The Mechanisms and Efficacy of Photobiomodulation Therapy for Arthritis: A Comprehensive Review', *International Journal of Molecular Sciences*, 24:18 (September 2023), https://doi.org/10.3390/ijms241814293

17 MT Sit et al, 'The Effects of Hyperbaric Oxygen on Rheumatoid Arthritis: A Pilot Study', *Journal of Clinical Rheumatology*, 1:27, 462–468 (December 2021), https://doi.org/10.1097/RHU.0000000000001540

18 D Alsina MBE, 'Driven by Experience, Powered by Change: Welcome to Arthritis UK', Arthritis UK (15 October 2025), www.arthritis-uk.org/news/2025/october/driven-by-experience-powered-by-change-welcome-to-arthritis-uk, accessed 12 March 2026

19 BR Deshpande et al, 'The number of persons with symptomatic knee osteoarthritis in the United States: Impact of race/ethnicity, age, sex, and obesity', *Arthritis Care & Research*, 68:12 (December 2016), https://doi.org/10.1002/acr.22897

20 JM Hootman et al, 'Updated Projected Prevalence of Self-Reported Doctor-Diagnosed Arthritis and Arthritis-Attributable Activity Limitation Among US Adults, 2015-2040', *Arthritis & Rheumatology*, 68:7 (July 2016), https://doi.org/10.1002/art.39692

21 S Swain, 'Trends in incidence and prevalence of osteoarthritis in the United Kingdom: findings from the Clinical Practice Research Datalink (CPRD)', *Osteoarthritis Cartilage*, 28:6, 792–801 (June 2020), https://doi.org/10.1016/j.joca.2020.03.004

22 E Alentorn-Geli et al, 'The Association of Recreational and Competitive Running With Hip and Knee Osteoarthritis: A Systematic Review and Meta-analysis', *Journal of Orthopaedic & Sports Physical Therapy*, 47:6 (June 2017), https://doi.org/10.2519/jospt.2017.7137

23 B Tayfur, C Charuphongsa et al, 'Neuromuscular joint function in knee osteoarthritis: A systematic review and meta-analysis', *Science Direct*, 66:2 (March 2023),

www.sciencedirect.com/science/article/pii/S1877065722000355, accessed 11 February 2026

24 T Nishimura, R Miyachi, 'Relationship between low back pain and lumbar and hip joint movement in desk workers', *Journal of Physical Therapy Science*, 32:10, 680–685 (3 October 2020), https://pmc.ncbi.nlm.nih.gov/articles/PMC7590845, accessed 11 February 2026

25 NICE, 'Management of osteoarthritis' (October 2022), www.nice.org.uk/guidance/ng226/resources/visual-summary-on-the-management-of-osteoarthritis-pdf-11251842157, accessed 11 February 2026

26 L Yan, D Li et al, 'Comparative efficacy and safety of exercise modalities in knee osteoarthritis: Systematic review and network meta-analysis', *BMJ* (15 October 2025), www.bmj.com/content/391/bmj-2025-085242, accessed 11 February 2026

27 T Moseng et al, 'EULAR recommendations for the non-pharmacological core management of hip and knee osteoarthritis: 2023 update', *Annals of the Rheumatic Diseases*, 83:6, 730–740 (2024), https://doi.org/10.1136/ard-2023-225041

28 S Sazo-Rodríguez et al, 'Effects of neuromuscular training on pain intensity, functionality, and quality of life in people with knee osteoarthritis: Systematic review with moderator analysis', *Physical Medicine and Rehabilitation* (6 November 2025), https://doi.org/10.1002/pmrj.70039

29 Ibid

30 AP Woodward, AM Fearon et al, 'Minimal clinically important change of knee flexion in people with knee osteoarthritis after non-surgical interventions using a meta-analytical approach', *Systematic Reviews*, 13:1, 50 (February 2024), https://pubmed.ncbi.nlm.nih.gov/38303000, accessed 11 February 2026

31 T Oka, O Wada et al, 'Importance of knee flexion range of motion during the acute phase after total knee arthroplasty', *Physiotherapy Theory and Practice*, 23:2, 143–148 (5 August 2020), https://pmc.ncbi.nlm.nih.gov/articles/PMC7814201, accessed 11 February 2026

32 MH El Gendy, MM Zalabia et al, 'Efficacy of rectus femoris stretching on pain, range of motion and spatiotemporal gait parameters in patients with knee osteoarthritis: a randomized controlled trial', *BMJ Open Sports & Exercise*

Medicine, 8:4 (December 2022), https://pmc.ncbi.nlm.nih.gov/articles/PMC9756178, accessed 11 February 2026

33 Z Tan, J Wang et al, 'Effects of heel kicking exercise on knee pain and joint function in knee osteoarthritis: A randomized controlled trial', *Medicine*, 104:16 (April 2025), https://pubmed.ncbi.nlm.nih.gov/40258742, accessed 11 February 2026

34 DT Thomas, C Eapen et al, 'Effectiveness of the core activation and rehabilitation exercises for knee osteoarthritis-program (CARE-KOA©) among patients diagnosed with knee osteoarthritis', *F1000Research*, 14:496 (July 2025), https://pubmed.ncbi.nlm.nih.gov/40799462, accessed 11 February 2026

35 A Gunn, TA Schwartz et al, 'Fear of Movement and Associated Factors Among Adults With Symptomatic Knee Osteoarthritis', *Arthritis Care & Research*, 69:12 (June 2018), https://pmc.ncbi.nlm.nih.gov/articles/PMC6020682, accessed 11 February 2026

36 J Lim, A Choi et al, 'The effects of resistance training on pain, strength, and function in osteoarthritis: Systematic review and meta-analysis', *Journal of Personalized Medicine*, 14:12 (30 November 2024), https://pmc.ncbi.nlm.nih.gov/articles/PMC11676110, accessed 11 February 2026

37 L Yan, D Li et al, 'Comparative efficacy and safety of exercise modalities in knee osteoarthritis: systematic review and network meta-analysis', *BMJ* (15 October 2025), www.bmj.com/content/391/bmj-2025-085242, accessed 11 February 2026

38 F Raposo, M Ramos, AL Cruz, 'Effects of exercise on knee osteoarthritis: A systematic review', *Musculoskeletal Care*, 19:4, 399–435 (December 2021), https://pubmed.ncbi.nlm.nih.gov/33666347, accessed 11 February 2026

39 KA Marriott, M Hall et al, 'Are the effects of resistance exercise on pain and function in knee and hip osteoarthritis dependent on exercise volume, duration, and adherence? A systematic review and meta-analysis', *ACR, Arthritis Care & Research*, 76:6, 821–830 (5 February 2024), https://acrjournals.onlinelibrary.wiley.com/doi/10.1002/acr.25313, accessed 11 February 2026

40 NIHR, 'People with osteoarthritis can benefit from exercise but may harbor myths about safety', *Muscle and Bone* (21 August 2018), https://evidence.nihr.ac.uk/alert/

people-with-osteoarthritis-can-benefit-from-exercise-but-may-harbour-myths-about-safety, accessed 11 February 2026
41 C-Y Zeng, Z-R Zhang, Z-M Tang, F-Z Hua, 'Benefits and mechanisms of exercise training for knee osteoarthritis, *Frontiers in Physiology*, 12, (16 December 2021), www.frontiersin.org/journals/physiology/articles/10.3389/fphys.2021.794062/full, accessed 11 February 2026
42 J Lim, A Choi et al, 'The effects of resistance training on pain, strength, and function in osteoarthritis: Systematic review and meta-analysis', *Journal of Personalized Medicine*, 14:12 (30 November 2024), https://pmc.ncbi.nlm.nih.gov/articles/PMC11676110, accessed 11 February 2026
43 L Yan, D Li et al, 'Comparative efficacy and safety of exercise modalities in knee osteoarthritis: Systematic review and network meta-analysis', *BMJ* (15 October 2025), www.bmj.com/content/391/bmj-2025-085242, accessed 11 February 2026
44 L Yan, D Li et al, 'Comparative efficacy and safety of exercise modalities in knee osteoarthritis: Systematic review and network meta-analysis', *BMJ* (15 October 2025), www.bmj.com/content/391/bmj-2025-085242, accessed 11 February 2026
45 A Money, A MacKenzie et al, 'Evidence on non-pharmacological interventions for preventing or reversing physical frailty in community-dwelling older adults over 50 years: overview of systematic reviews', *BMC Geriatrics*, 25:183 (17 March 2025), https://pmc.ncbi.nlm.nih.gov/articles/PMC11912688, accessed 11 February 2026
46 S Messier, DJ Gutekunst et al, 'Weight loss reduces knee-joint loads in overweight and obese older adults with knee osteoarthritis', *Arthritis & Rheumatology*, 52:7 (July 2005), https://pubmed.ncbi.nlm.nih.gov/15986358, accessed 11 February 2026
47 SP Messier, DP Beavers, K Queen, 'Effect of diet and exercise on knee pain in patients with osteoarthritis and overweight or obesity: A randomized clinical trial', *JAMA Networks*, 328:2 (13 December 2022), https://jamanetwork.com/journals/jama/fullarticle/2799405, accessed 11 February 2026
48 X Ma, F Nan et al, 'Excessive intake of sugar: An accomplice of inflammation', *Frontiers in Immunology* (31 August 2022), https://pmc.ncbi.nlm.nih.gov/articles/PMC9471313, accessed 11 February 2026

49 JC Maroon, JW Bost, 'Omega-3 fatty acids (fish oil) as an anti-inflammatory: an alternative to nonsteroidal anti-inflammatory drugs for discogenic pain', *Surgical Neurology*, 65:4, 326–31 (April 2006), https://pubmed.ncbi.nlm.nih.gov/16531187, accessed 11 February 2026
50 JW Daily, M Yang, S Park, 'Efficacy of turmeric extracts and curcumin for alleviating the symptoms of joint arthritis: A systematic review and meta-analysis of randomized clinical trials', *Journal of Medicinal Food*, 19:8, 717–729 (1 August 2016), https://pmc.ncbi.nlm.nih.gov/articles/PMC5003001, accessed 11 February 2026
51 JW Daily, M Yang, S Park, 'Efficacy of turmeric extracts and curcumin for alleviating the symptoms of joint arthritis: A systematic review and meta-analysis of randomized clinical trials', *Journal of Medicinal Food*, 19:8, 717–729 (1 August 2016), https://pmc.ncbi.nlm.nih.gov/articles/PMC5003001, accessed 11 February 2026
52 RR Bannuru, MC Osani, F Al Eid, C Wang, 'Efficacy of curcumin and boswellia for knee osteoarthritis: Systematic review and meta-analysis', *Seminars in Arthritis and Rheumatism* (1 December 2019), https://pmc.ncbi.nlm.nih.gov/articles/PMC6131088, accessed 11 February 2026
53 K Elgar, 'EPA/DHA: A Review of Clinical Use and Efficacy', *Nutritional Medicine Journal*, 1:2, 97–132 (2022), www.nmi.health/epa-dha-a-review-of-clinical-use-and-efficacy, accessed 12 March 2026
54 JM Garcia-Coronado, L Martinez-Olvera et al, 'Effect of collagen supplementation on osteoarthritis symptoms: A meta-analysis of randomized placebo-controlled trials', *International Orthopaedics*, 43:3, 531–538 (March 2019), https://pubmed.ncbi.nlm.nih.gov/30368550, accessed 13 February 2026
55 PJ Brueckheimer, TC Silva et al, 'The effects of type 1 collagen hydrolysate supplementation on bones, muscles, and joints: A systematic review', *Orthopedic Reviews* (PDF), 17 (2025), https://orthopedicreviews.openmedicalpublishing.org/api/v1/articles/129086-the-effects-of-type-i-collagen-hydrolysate-supplementation-on-bones-muscles-and-joints-a-systematic-review.pdf, accessed 13 February 2026
56 LM Hengeveld, JMA Boer et al, 'Prevalence of protein intake below recommended in community-dwelling older adults: a meta-analysis across cohorts from the PROMISS

consortium', *Journal of Cachexia, Sarcopenia and Muscle*, 11:5, 1211222 (October 2020), https://pubmed.ncbi.nlm.nih.gov/32548960, accessed 13 February 2026

57 RW Morton, KT Murphy et al, 'A systematic review, meta-analysis and meta-regression of the effect of protein supplementation on resistance training-induced gains in muscle mass and strength in healthy adults', *BMJ Journals*, 52:6 (1 Oct 2020), https://bjsm.bmj.com/content/52/6/376, accessed 13 February 2026

58 MC Devries, SM Phillips, 'Creatine supplementation during resistance training in older adults–a meta-analysis', *Medicine & Science in Sports & Exercise*, 46:6, 1194–203 (June 2014), https://pubmed.ncbi.nlm.nih.gov/24576864, accessed 13 February 2026

59 A Gordji-Nejad et al, 'Single dose creatine improves cognitive performance and induces changes in cerebral high energy phosphates during sleep deprivation', *Scientific Reports*, 14:4937 (2024), https://doi.org/10.1038/s41598-024-54249-9

60 A Rabade, GL Viswanatha et al, 'Evaluation of efficacy and safety of glucosamine sulfate, chondroitin sulfate, and their combination regimen in the management of knee osteoarthritis: a systematic review and meta-analysis', *Inflammopharmacology*, 32:3, 1759–1775 (June 2024), https://pubmed.ncbi.nlm.nih.gov/38581640, accessed 13 February 2026

61 N Veronese, FS Ragusa et al, 'Mediterranean diet and osteoarthritis: An update', *Aging Clinical and Experimental Research*, 36:1, 231 (3 December 2024), https://pmc.ncbi.nlm.nih.gov/articles/PMC11614952, accessed 13 February 2026

62 AJ Krause, AA Prather et al, 'The pain of sleep loss: A brain characterization in humans', *Journal of Neuroscience*, 39:12, 2291–2300 (20 March 2019), https://pubmed.ncbi.nlm.nih.gov/30692228, accessed 13 February 2026

63 LB Baker, M Ozga et al, 'Mild dehydration does not alter acute changes in sweat electrolyte concentrations during exercise', *Physiological Reports*, 12:18, e16174 (18 September 2024), https://pmc.ncbi.nlm.nih.gov/articles/PMC11410553, accessed 13 February 2026

64 F Roggio, L Petrigna et al, 'The role of lubricin, irisin and exercise in the prevention and treatment of osteoarthritis', *International Journal of Molecular Sciences*, 24:6, 5126

(7 March 2023), https://pmc.ncbi.nlm.nih.gov/articles/PMC10049370, accessed 13 February 2026

65 E-J Kim, JE Dimsdale, 'The effect of psychosocial stress on sleep: A review of polysomnographic evidence', *Behavioral Sleep Medicine*, 5:4, 256–278 (2007), https://pmc.ncbi.nlm.nih.gov/articles/PMC4266573, accessed 13 February 2026

66 AM González-Roldán et al, 'Age-Related Changes in Pain Perception Are Associated With Altered Functional Connectivity During Resting State', *Frontiers in Aging Neuroscience*, 12:116, https://doi.org/10.3389/fnagi.2020.00116

67 M Choueiri, X Chevalier, F Eymard, 'Intraarticular Corticosteroids for Hip Osteoarthritis: A Review', *Cartilage*, 13:1 (Suppl), 122S–131S (20 August 2020), https://pmc.ncbi.nlm.nih.gov/articles/PMC8808783, accessed 13 February 2026

68 TE McAlindon et al, 'Effect of Intra-articular Triamcinolone vs Saline on Knee Cartilage Volume and Pain in Patients With Knee Osteoarthritis: A Randomized Clinical Trial', *The Journal of the American Medical Association*, 16:317 (May 2017), https://doi.org/10.1001/jama.2017.5283

69 S Ayub et al, 'Efficacy and safety of multiple intra-articular corticosteroid injections for osteoarthritis–a systematic review and meta-analysis of randomized controlled trials and observational studies', *Rheumatology*, 6:60 (April 2021), https://doi.org/10.1093/rheumatology/keaa808

70 TV Pereira et al, 'Viscosupplementation for knee osteoarthritis: systematic review and meta-analysis', *British Medical Journal*, 378:e069722 (July 2022), https://doi.org/10.1136/bmj-2022-069722

71 EN Bowman, JD Hallock, TW Throckmorton and FM Azar, 'Hyaluronic acid injections for osteoarthritis of the knee: predictors of successful treatment', *International Orthopaedics*, 42:4, 733–740 (April 2018), https://doi.org/10.1007/s00264-017-3731-8

72 D-M Ellingsen, V Napadow et al, 'Brain mechanisms of anticipated painful movements and their modulation by manual therapy in chronic low back pain', *The Journal of Pain* (1 November 2019), https://pmc.ncbi.nlm.nih.gov/articles/PMC6220681, accessed 13 February 2026

73 M Poulain, 'Exceptional longevity in Okinawa: Demographic trends since 1975', *Journal of Internal Medicine*

(14 January 2024), https://onlinelibrary.wiley.com/doi/10.1111/joim.13764, accessed 6 February 2026

74 Geneva, 'Social connection linked to improved health and reduced risk of early death' (World Health Organization, 30 June 2025), www.who.int/news/item/30-06-2025-social-connection-linked-to-improved-heath-and-reduced-risk-of-early-death, accessed 6 February 2026

75 T Laukkanen, JA Laukkanen, H Khan and F Zaccardi, 'Association between sauna bathing and fatal cardiovascular and all-cause mortality events', *Journal of American Medical Association*, 175:4, 542–548 (April 2015), https://doi.org/10.1001/jamainternmed.2014.8187

76 R Zhang and J Qu, 'The Mechanisms and Efficacy of Photobiomodulation therapy for Arthritis: A Comprehensive Review', *International Journal of Molecular Science*, 24:18 (September 2023), https://doi.org/10.3390/ijms241814293

77 E Vasenina et al, 'The acute muscular response following a novel form of pulsed direct current stimulation (Neubie) or traditional resistance exercise', *Journal of Musculoskeletal and Neuronal Interactions*, 22:3, 336–345 (September 2022), https://pubmed.ncbi.nlm.nih.gov/36046989, accessed 12 March 2026

78 NeuFit, 'Case Study' (n.d), www.neu.fit/wp-content/uploads/2024/07/24-Year-Old-NFL-Running-Back-With-ACLMCL-Reconstruction-And-Meniscus-Tear-Repair-A-Case-Study-Report.pdf, accessed 13 March 2026

Resources

I've put together a simple online hub I call the Vault. You'll find guided exercise videos and movement examples that show you exactly how things should looks and feel. You can access the Vault at pages.philthephysio.com/vault or by scanning the QR code below:

You can take the health questionnaire by visiting quiz.philthephysio.com/start-here or by scanning the QR code below:

Acknowledgements

Although there is one name on the cover, this book has been shaped by thousands of people over many years.

First and foremost, thank you to the patients I have worked with throughout my career. Many of the lessons in these pages come directly from real conversations, real frustrations, and real progress seen in clinic every week. Your willingness to stay consistent, even when progress feels slow, continually reinforces what the human body is capable of at any age. It has been a privilege to support so many people in regaining confidence in their movement and returning to the activities that make life enjoyable.

Thank you to the team at Urban Body. The care, professionalism, and attention you give every person who walks through the door is what allows these principles to work in the real world, not just on paper. The results people achieve are built on the standards you deliver every single day. A special thank you to Karen, who has been instrumental in building Urban Body into what it is today. Your commitment to maintaining the highest standards across everything we do, and your dedication to the clinic and everything it stands for, gave me the freedom to write this book without ever having to worry about what was happening behind me. That trust is not something I take lightly.

To the mentors, teachers, and colleagues who shaped how I think about movement, rehabilitation, and long-term health, thank you. A special mention to the late Paula Wilde, who treated me as a child and unknowingly inspired me to become a physio, and to Eileen Taylor, whose mentorship throughout my time at Loughborough University gave me the foundations everything in this book is built on.

Thank you to Mike and the team at Rethink Press for helping bring this book to life and guiding it from idea to finished manuscript.

To my parents, thank you for setting the standard long before this book was written. Your support throughout my career, from the very beginning when Urban Body started in your front room, to everything that has followed since, has meant the world to me. You never told me that growing older meant slowing down; you just never did. Watching you run around with my children – keeping up with their energy, playing, laughing, and fully taking part in their lives – is one of the true joys of my life. That doesn't happen by accident. It is built through years of valuing your health, staying consistent with movement, and respecting what your body allows you to do. You have lived everything this book stands for, and I am grateful for that every day.

To my partner, Steph. Twelve years together, three children – Sydney, Hugo, and Max – and a vision that has not always been easy to follow. You have held our family together through all of it, without ever questioning where this was heading. You have been my biggest believer from the very beginning, whether that was in the early days of Urban Body, through the late evenings building something we believed in, or sitting with each chapter of this book as it developed and helping me find the right words. That belief has meant more than I can properly put into words. None of this would exist without you.

Finally, thank you to you, the reader. Choosing to take responsibility for your health is not always easy, particularly when advice can feel confusing or progress slower than expected. The decision to build strength, maintain independence, and stay engaged in your own wellbeing is one that pays dividends for years to come.

Phil

The Author

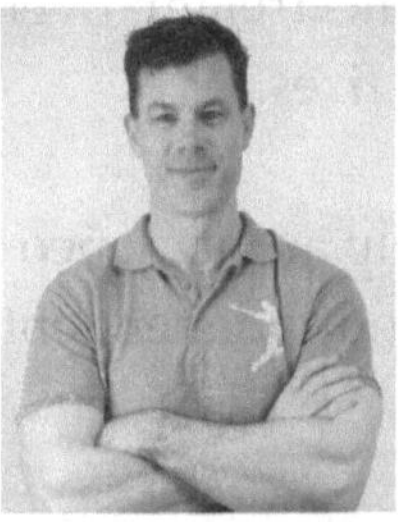

Phil Evans is a chartered physiotherapist with twenty years' experience of helping people move better, get stronger, and stay independent as they age.

He began his career working in elite sport, supporting professional rugby players, international cricketers, and Olympic and Commonwealth athletes, where performance and long-term resilience were non-negotiable. If an athlete couldn't move well, they couldn't compete. Simple as that.

Alongside that world, Phil saw a very different reality playing out every day in general healthcare. People over fifty with joint pain, stiffness, or arthritis were often given painkillers, vague advice, or long waits for surgery, with little explanation and even less confidence. The contrast frustrated him.

That gap is why Phil founded Urban Body, a physiotherapy clinic based in Solihull, UK. There, he and his team work primarily with adults over fifty who want to stay active, capable, and independent. The clinic combines straightforward evidence-based physiotherapy with advanced rehabilitation technologies traditionally reserved for elite sport, always guided by what helps people move and live better in the real world.

This book reflects the same principles Phil uses in clinic every day: clarity over confusion, strength over fear, and sensible progress over quick fixes.

His aim has always been simple: to help as many people as possible stay strong, mobile, and independent as they get older.

You can find out more about Phil and his work at:

- www.urbanbody.co.uk
- www.philthephysio.com
- @philthephysio

www.ingramcontent.com/pod-product-compliance
Lightning Source LLC
LaVergne TN
LVHW040517210926
848480LV00007BA/1498